MYTHS, MISCONCEPTIONS, AND HEROICS
THE STORY OF THE TREATMENT OF
HYPERTENSION FROM THE 1930s

Marvin Moser, MD
Clinical Professor of Medicine,
Yale University School of Medicine
Senior Medical Consultant
National High Blood Pressure Education Program
National Heart, Lung and Blood Institute

In commemoration of the 25th Anniversary of the National
High Blood Pressure Education Program 1997

Le Jacq Communications, Inc.
1997

ISBN: 0-9626020-4-3

Printed in the United States of America

INTRODUCTION

1997 marks the 25th anniversary of the establishment of the National High Blood Pressure Education Program (NHBPEP). This program has been labeled one of the most successful in preventive medicine in the U.S. in the past 50 years. This monograph is written in commemoration of the achievements of the NHBPEP over the past 25 years. It reviews some of the misconceptions and myths about hypertension that were and still are prevalent. It describes some of the heroic measures undertaken in the 1930s–1950s by physicians who refused to believe the then current teachings that elevated blood pressure was a natural adaptive mechanism necessary to increase blood flow to various organs as people aged. These were the physicians who recognized that lowering blood pressure might be beneficial. The tools that they had to work with were primitive and included mutilative surgery, rigid and impossible-to-follow dietary restrictions, or the injection of fever producing pyrogens. Their efforts were indeed heroic. Fortunately, with the evolution of effective antihypertensive medication and a better understanding of lifestyle modifications that may help to lower blood pressure, we have advanced to a time in 1997 when a great majority of hypertensive patients can have their blood pressure lowered successfully and can lead normal and enjoyable lives without restrictions.

We still have a long way to go and many things to learn about the more effective use of the tools we have at hand, but we have clarified many of the misconceptions and myths and replaced heroics with rational, reasonable approaches as we commemorate this important anniversary.

The NHBPEP was established in 1972 by the National Heart, Lung & Blood Institute (NHLBI) as part of a national effort to improve the control of hypertension. The program was designed to: 1) bring together physicians and other health care personnel involved in the detection and control of hypertension; 2) gather all available information on the etiology, prevention, diagnosis, and treatment of hypertension; and 3) disseminate this information as widely as possible to both the general public and health care personnel. Its mission was: 1) to increase the numbers of patients who were aware of their elevated blood pressure; 2) to alert the public to the dangers of even slightly elevated blood pressure; 3) to redefine levels of blood pressure that were of significance and that should be evaluated and treated; 4) to review various therapies and suggest guidelines for treatment; and, finally and most importantly 5) to reduce morbidity and mortality that may result from hypertension.

Over the past 25 years, this organization, guided by the National High Blood Pressure Coordinating Committee, under the leadership of the Director of the NHLBI, has issued position papers dealing with the diagnostic evaluation, and treatment of hypertension, kidney disease and hypertension, hypertension and pregnancy, hypertension in children, and lifestyle modifications for primary prevention or treatment of high blood pressure. In addition, an active public education effort, with support from the pharmaceutical industry, has helped to increase the public's awareness of hypertension and the numbers of hypertensive patients who are being effectively treated. The cornerstone of the NHBPEP has been the Joint National Committee Reports on the Detection, Evaluation and Treatment of High Blood Pressure (JNC). These reports have been released approximately every 4 years and many of their recommendations have been accepted worldwide.

There are many participants in the story of hypertension treatment; it is impossible to mention them all. A few who were prominently involved in the NHBPEP in its first 10 years include Drs. Ted Cooper and Bob Levy, Mary Lasker, Elliot Richardson, and Graham Ward. Dr. Claude Lenfant, Director of the NHLBI, and Dr. Edward Roccella, Coordinator of the program, have led the Institute's program for more than a decade. Clinicians and researchers who have had an impact on defining both mechanisms and approaches to therapy include Drs. Irvine Page, Herbert Langford, Walter Kirkendall, Harriet Dustan, Edward Frohlich, Edward Freis, Jerimiah Stamler, William McFate Smith, Ray Gifford, Norman Kaplan, Lou Tobian, Susanne Oparil, John Laragh, Arthur Grollman, Harry Goldblatt, Mitchell Perry, Henry Schroeder, Alvin Shapiro, John Moyer, Joseph Wilbur, Harry Gavras, Aran Chobanian, Paul Whelton, Jeff Cutler, Myron Weinberger, Michael Weber, Charles Francis, James Sowers, Sheldon Sheps, Michael Alderman, Charles Curry, Henry Black, Martha Hill, Richard Grimm, and Michael Horan. Numerous other physicians and nurses have made significant contributions in many areas in the management of this disease.

My own involvement in the NHBPEP began with the Arlie House Conferences where physicians and other health care providers with an interest in hypertension were brought together to chart the course of a national program. I became the Senior Medical Consultant to the NHBPEP in 1974, was Chairman of the first JNC in 1977, and have actively participated in the program since that time. It is with some personal pride that I record some of the myths, misconceptions, and heroics in the management of hypertension in the last half of the 20th century and during the lifetime of the NHBPEP.

Marvin Moser, MD

> The aim of science is not to open a door
> to endless wisdom, but to put a limit to
> endless error.

Bertold Brecht: *The Life of Galileo*

Widespread Misconceptions

There are few stories in the history of medicine that are filled
with more errors or misconceptions than the story of hypertension and its treatment. It is not the purpose of this monograph
to review all of these but to highlight the changes in concept
and approach that have occurred in the latter part of the 20th
century—long after it had been recognized that elevated blood
pressure was not always preceded by kidney disease and that
bleeding with leeches or venosection were not always the best
approach to treatment. As late as the 1930s misconceptions
were common.

In 1931 Dr. Paul Dudley White, an eminent Boston cardiolo-
gist, wrote that "Hypertension may be an important compensatory
mechanism which should not be tampered with, even were it certain that we could control it," and Hay, in the *British Medical
Journal* (1931;2:43–47) stated that:

> The greatest danger to a man with high
> blood pressure lies in its discovery,
> because then some fool is certain to try
> and reduce it.

The concept that hypertension was an essential adaptive reaction may have arisen because of the original designation of hypertension as "hypertonie essential"—essential hypertension. This
belief persisted for many years and probably contributed to the
delay in acknowledging the significance of hypertension as an
abnormal phenomenon. It also served to discourage any attempts
to lower blood pressure. This still appears to have been the belief
of many physicians throughout the 1940s. Scott, in the 1946 edition of Tice's *Practice of Medicine*, one of the leading textbooks
of medicine at the time, advised:

> "May not the elevation of systemic blood

pressure be a natural response to guarantee
a more normal circulation to the heart,
brain and kidneys" ("essential" hypertension)
and commented that:

"Overzealous attempts to lower the pressure
may do no good and often do harm." or that
"Many cases of essential hypertension not
only do not need any treatment but are much
better off without it. Generally the less
said about the blood pressure in such people,
the better"[1]

The press was sending confusing messages to the public. A
San Francisco newspaper in 1949 declared:

Scientists fight high blood pressure, the
greatest killer of the middle aged.

Yet at the same time a monthly digest magazine proclaimed:

High Blood Pressure? Don't be alarmed—when
the facts become known, a brooding and paralyzing
fear should lift from the land.

Obviously, science writers as well as physicians were confused.

Early Attempts at Treatment

It was within this climate of confusion, and despite pronouncements of leading cardiologists that some physicians recognized
the dangers of high blood pressure and began to explore methods
of lowering it. Treatments, although well intentioned, were often
bizarre and harmful. Weiss in *1939*[2] summarized the state of the
art of therapy and elaborated on some of the mistaken theories
that determined the types of treatment offered:

Thus far, what has been done in an effort
to reduce the blood pressure? Because of
an ill-founded idea that protein was
responsible for hypertension and kidney

disease the patient was denied meat and eggs, and especially red meat...His diet was rendered even more unpalatable by the withdrawal of salt.

Reduction of fat and cholesterol intake was suggested for the wrong reasons—the concept in the 1920's and 1930's (that a high protein intake induced kidney disease which caused hypertension). But this was not bad advice. A high salt intake had been associated with a "hard pulse," high blood pressure, and strokes for many years—this also appeared to be good advice. But, Weiss continued:

Sympathy would doubtless have been extended to this half-starved fellow except that he probably was not able to eat anyway, his teeth having been extracted on the theory that focal infection had something to do with hypertension. Even before this he had sacrificed his tonsils and had had his sinuses punctured because of the same theory. In case some food has been consumed, the slight colonic residue was promptly washed out by numerous colonic irrigations, especially during the period when the theory of autointoxication was enjoying a wave of popularity.

To add to his unhappiness he was often told to stop work. Of course, he was denied coffee and tea, and as a climax to the difficulties of this unfortunate person, he may now fall into the clutches of the neurosurgeon, who is prepared to separate him from his sympathetic nervous system.

Attempts at lowering blood pressure were often based on poor science or desperation, and the cause of elevated blood pressure was not known in more than 90% of patients. An obvious question at that time was—how can we treat a disease when we do not know its cause?

Table I. FDR—A Case of Untreated Hypertension			
Year	Blood Pressure (mm Hg)	Complications	Treatment
1935	136/78—age 53		
1937	162/98		Phenobarbitol
1937–1941	170–180/90–100		Low-salt and low-fat diet Massages 1941
	188/105	Cardiac enlargement	
		Probable lacunar infarcts	
1944	186/108	{ Congestive heart failure	Digitalis
1944–1945	180–230/110–126	Renal failure	
April 12, 1945—cerebral hemorrhage—death, age 63			

A Case of Untreated Hypertension

A typical case of untreated hypertension in the 1940s was that of Franklin Delano Roosevelt whose blood pressure became elevated in 1937 and progressively rose from levels of 160/90 mm Hg to levels of 220–230/140–150 mm Hg over the next 7–8 years.[3] We must remember that he lived in an era when effective treatment was not available and when many physicians were still not convinced that hypertension resulted in vascular injury or that lowering it would be effective. It is well documented that he developed left ventricular hypertrophy (LVH), multiple lacunar infarcts, and in 1944, congestive heart failure (CHF), and renal failure. He died at a relatively young age of 63 of cerebral hemorrhage. His treatment had variously consisted of phenobarbital, a low-fat, low-sodium diet, and rest (Table I). No other therapy was suggested. Of course, the President was also a heavy smoker, which may also have contributed to his progressive illness.

Roosevelt's symptoms were often misdiagnosed. For example, during his last year of life when he experienced extreme fatigue and paroxysmal nocturnal dyspnea as well as marked shortness of breath on minimal activity, his physician advised that this was due to recurrent bronchitis, allergies, or the flu. It was only after the intervention of Mrs. Roosevelt's daughter, who had come to live at the White House, that another physician was called in to see the president. A diagnosis of CHF was made. When it was suggested that definitive treatment, which included digitalis, be given to the President, this was carried out reluctantly since his personal physician was concerned about "frightening" the public. Had Roosevelt lived 20 years later, he might have been treated effectively and many of the complications that occurred would have been delayed or prevented.

> A little fire is quickly trodden out; which,
> being suffered, rivers cannot quench.

This quote from Shakespeare's King Henry VI suggests an approach to management which, while almost impossible to carry out prior to the early 1950s, became easier to implement as the years progressed: The treatment of hypertension at an early stage *will* quench the little fire before it spreads. This is the approach that some heroic investigators and clinicians attempted in the years following Roosevelt's death.

The Beginnings of Diet, Surgical, and Drug Therapy

The late 1940s and 1950s heralded a dramatic change in the approach to the treatment of hypertension. While there were still some physicians who continued to have doubts regarding the significance of hypertension, most had accepted the fact that elevated blood pressure was not necessary to profuse organs and that increased pressure increased risk for cardiovascular disease. In addition, there were now some data that, at least in severe, accelerated, or malignant hypertension, suggested the lowering of blood pressure reversed some of the complications of the disease. We had learned from the experience of Kempner that a rigid low-sodium diet, which consisted mostly of fruit, fruit juice, and rice, and contained just 20 g of protein, only 5 g of fat, and less than 200 mg of sodium, could reduce the complications of malignant hypertension; papilledema cleared in some patients and heart failure was improved.[4] Although Sir George Pickering, a physician-philosopher in Great Britain, described the diet as "insipid, unappetizing, monotonous, unacceptable, and intolerable," and that to stay on it "required the ascetism of a religious zealot," a few people did respond and were able to stay on the diet long enough for an effect to be noticed. Considering that the prognosis of malignant hypertension was worse than many cancerous lesions with death within 6 months to 1 year in untreated cases,[5,6] this approach, although impractical for most people, did help some. In 1948 Kempner reported that 322 of 500 patients had improved on this program.[4]

In addition to studies on dietary restriction, data had been accumulated indicating that extensive interruption of the sympathetic nervous system, with or without adrenalectomy, could also temporarily halt the progression of severe hypertension in as many as 40%–50% of patients.[7,8] But at what a price! Patients were frequently hospitalized for 6–8 weeks, postoperative complications were often severe with marked postural hypotension and syncope, impotence, and lack of sweating. In many cases the use of pressure suits was necessary for patients to be able to ambulate. The preoperative evaluation was of interest. Intravenous sodium amytal was given. If blood pressures did not decrease significantly, it was considered that the disease was not severe enough to warrant surgical therapy or that there would be little or no response to surgery. Surgical therapy was undertaken if the "semicomatose" patient's blood pressure was reduced to normal. Even this "dramatic" test, as with many others, was not always predictive. In subjects whose adrenal glands were removed, replacement hormones had to be given. These procedures were probably justified, however, in patients with true malignant hypertension, with a 3–6 month life expectancy.

Experience with sympathectomies laid the groundwork for the development of medications that effectively blocked the sympathetic nervous system—phentolamine, phenoxybenzamine, or the ganglion blocking agents, etc., but other attempts to lower blood pressure were also being tried.

In the 1940s, Drs. Freis and Page resorted to vasodilation treatment in patients with malignant hypertension. Freis commented, after using pentaquine, that:

> This was the first time we had seen reversal
> of the signs of malignant hypertension
> following an antihypertensive drug. It was
> an exciting experience.[9]

And Page, in 1949, after trying pyrogen injections with some success, stated that:

> I need hardly say this is an unpleasant treatment but considering the danger of the disease to the life of the patient it is a small price to pay for the benefits.[10]

But benefits didn't persist for long.

The Early Medications

Rauwolfia Drugs

We also had had some experience with various more specific antihypertensive drugs in the late 1940s and early 1950s (Table II). In the early 1950s, the rauwolfia compounds were introduced in the U.S. These drugs had been used for centuries in India and elsewhere as sedatives and were effective catecholamine depletors, both centrally and peripherally. Initial experience suggested

---

Table II. Available Antihypertensive Drugs From the 1930s to the 1990s

1930s	Veratrum alkaloids
1940s	Thiocyanates
	Ganglion blocking agents
	Catecholamine depletors (Rauwolfia derivatives)
1950s	Vasodilators (Hydralazine)
	Peripheral sympathetic inhibitors (Guanethidine)
	(Phenoxybenzamine)
	Monamine oxidase inhibitors
	Diuretics
	Combinations of diuretics and other medications
1960s	Central α_2 agonists
	(sympathetic nervous system inhibitors)
	ß-Adrenergic inhibitors
1970	α-Adrenergic inhibitors
	α-ß-Blockers
	Converting enzyme inhibitors
1980s	Calcium channel blockers
1990s	Angiotensin II receptor antagonists

that approximately 20% of patients would show a response when they were used as monotherapy.[11,12] The Committee on Chemotherapy and Hypertension of the Council for High Blood Pressure Research of the American Heart Association agreed in 1957 that some form of rauwolfia derivative was the drug of choice with which to begin antihypertensive treatment. This class of drugs produced better blood pressure lowering results than sedatives such as phenobarbital. The literature noted that perhaps in our "charged up Westernized Society," a little bit of sedation or slowing down might be a good thing, especially if it helped to lower blood pressure. When a rauwolfia derivative was given in combination with a thiazide diuretic (in the late 1950s) a high percentage of patients (as many as 80% in some series) became normotensive. The rauwolfia drugs were and are inexpensive, effective in a once-a-day dosage, and produce no metabolic changes or deleterious hemodynamic effects. Some serious depressions, as well as fatigue and insomnia were, however, reported following the use of these medications, especially when given in dosages of more than 0.5 mg per day; depressions often persisted for 4 to 6 weeks or more after the drug was stopped. Many of us used dosages as high as 1 or 2 mg per day and, in cases of hypertensive encephalopathy, as much as 5 to 10 mg was often administered intramuscularly. As more was learned about these medications and lower dosages were used, depression became a less frequent occurrence, although this reaction is still noted occasionally. It is often subtle and difficult to diagnose early. In my judgement, rauwolfia drugs, in small dosages of 0.05 to 0.1 mg/gd, in combination with a diuretic agent, still have a place in hypertensive management, although they are rarely used at the present time.

Thiocyanates, Veratrum Derivatives, and Hydralazine

The *thiocyanates* also lowered blood pressure but the therapeutic and toxic doses were close, making therapy difficult to control.[13]

The *veratrum derivatives* acted by blocking vagal and baroreceptor impulses and were effective as antihypertensive drugs. However, here too, one dose might produce a slight lowering of blood pressure, whereas, an additional small increase in dosage might produce nausea, vomiting, severe dizziness, or syncope.[14] At one time these agents were widely used in the treatment of hypertension and toxemia of pregnancy.

Hydralazine, a potent vasodilator also lowered blood pressure effectively, but tolerance often developed and side effects such as tachycardia or headaches were common; in large doses (> 300–400 mg/day) a lupus-like syndrome occasionally developed.[15,16] This agent, when combined with other medications proved to be effective treatment in many patients during the 1960s.

It was recognized even then that only approximately 50% of patients responded to any one drug as monotherapy. This is true today despite the availability of newer and better tolerated medications.

In 1949–1950 we began working with phenoxybenzamine, a sympathetic blocking agent which blocked both pre- and postsympathetic ganglia. This agent produced a progressive, selective blockade of various parts of the sympathetic nervous system—a chemical sympathectomy with vasodilation in numerous vascular beds.[17] Vascular responses to norepinephrine were blocked, but norepinephrine reuptake was also prevented. Tachycardia and tachyphylaxis resulted and symptoms of dizziness and syncope were common. This agent subsequently proved to be an ineffective antihypertensive medication, and today it is mainly used with or without a ß-adrenergic inhibitor in the preoperative management of patients with pheochromocytoma. However, in the early 1950s it was an important compound to study because of its dramatic effect on the sympathetic nervous system.

Antihypertensive drug research, as well as research in other areas, was accelerating in the early 1950s—the national priorities for antibiotics during World War II were being replaced by a search for better medications to treat or prevent heart disease and other illnesses.

It is of interest to note that phenoxybenzamine was listed as Number "688A" at Smith Kline and French (now SmithKline Beecham) when it was first being studied in the late 1940s and early 1950s. Between that time and the present, more than 110,000 compounds have been evaluated by the same company for the treatment of various diseases—a commentary on the explosion of drug research since the end of World War II

The Ganglion and Peripheral Blocking Agents

We had also had some experience with the ganglion blocking agents—hexamethonium, pentolinium, mecamylamine, and a peripheral adrenergic inhibitor guanethidine.[18,19] These drugs were potent and highly effective as blood pressure lowering agents in many cases but, as was the case with many of the other available medications, their use resulted in significant side effects. The ganglion blockers not only produced what amounted to a chemical sympathectomy but also blocked the activity of the parasympathetic nervous system. Effect was often erratic and at first these medications had to be given by injection 3–4 times a day.[20]

Orally effective ganglion blockers did become available but absorption was erratic. Because of bowel atony and severe constipation in many individuals, a dosage given at 8:00 am might not be absorbed until 2:00 or 3:00 in the afternoon following the second dose given at noon. Collapse was not infrequent, as well as dry mouth, blurring of vision, severe constipation, and sexual dysfunction (actually these agents, as well as phenoxybenzamine, were effective male contraceptives—ejaculation was often prevented). When given in combination with reserpine and hydralazine, the ganglion blocking agents reduced blood pressure in a high percentage of patients who, if they could tolerate the medication, did reasonably well for long periods of time.

Thinking back to this era one might wonder how anyone could stay on therapy with 3 or 4 injections a day with a ganglion blocker or on many of the medications or combinations we were using. But, that was the only available therapy, and if a patient were symptomatic with heart failure or severe retinopathy and wished to survive, he or she put up with this type of complicated regimen. Freis[21,22] and Schroeder,[23] pioneers in the treatment of hypertension, combined the use of ganglion blockers, vasodilators, and catecholamine-depleting medications as Hyphex (hexamethonium and hydralazine) and Hypotensen A, B & C (various doses of a ganglion blocker [pentolinium], hydralazine, and reserpine).

Figure 1 illustrates a case of severe hypertension that initially did not respond to reserpine (Serpasil) and hydralazine (Apresoline). When a ganglion blocking agent, pentolinium (Ansolysen), was added to therapy in November 1954, blood pressures were reduced to a greater degree but not to consistently normotensive levels of < 140/90 mm Hg. Left ventricular hypertrophy regressed. Ganglion blocking agents were discontinued in 1959 and hydrochlorothiazide (HCTZ) was given. The patient survived for 7 years. A better result could probably have been

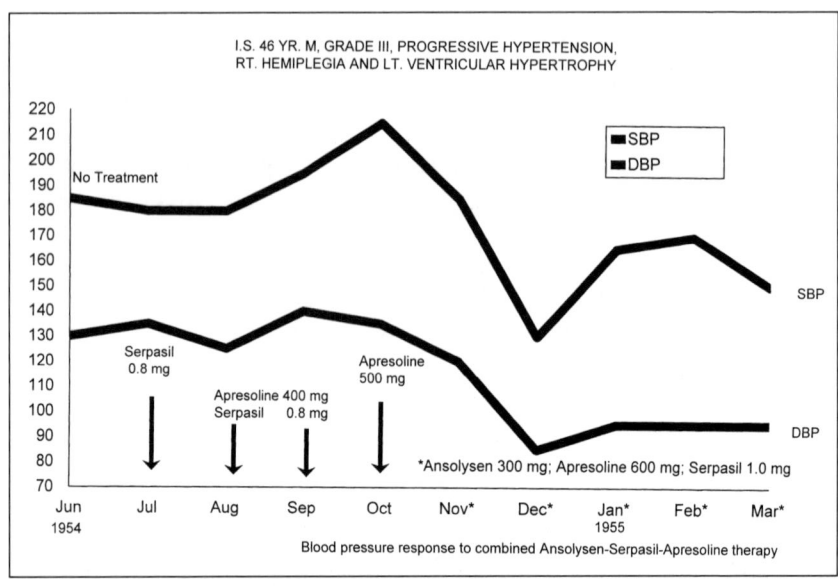

Figure 1. Example of a reasonably satisfactory blood pressure response after a ganglion blocker was added to vasodilator and catecholamine depletor therapy.

achieved with therapy that was better tolerated.

Because of the problems with drug therapy and the fact that few outcome data from controlled long-term trials were available, it was appropriate that only patients with severe hypertension were treated. In fact—*a recurrent theme that would not go away*—there were still many eminent physicians in the late 1950s who advised that hypertension need not be treated, that complications were inevitable, and there was little that could be done to prevent them—and we still did not know the cause of hypertension in more than 90% of patients.

1955—The Concept of "Benign" Hypertension Persists

In an oft quoted paper, Perrara estimated that the life expectancy of the hypertensive patient was approximately 52 years.[24] When untreated the condition appeared to run a course of about 20 years from the time of discovery, with few symptoms or complications for the first 10 years in most patients. It was only after this time that complications became more frequent. Prognosis was worse in males, especially in young males. Half of the patients untreated died of CHF, about 20% of vascular accidents, and 20% of uremia. (In other series, cerebrovascular accidents accounted for a higher percentage of mortality). The conclusions of this study were often accepted by physicians as indicating the "benign" nature of hypertension, but considering the fact that the average age of patients when follow-up was begun was in the 30s, the study strongly indicated a reason for early therapy. It is of interest to note that in the 1990s CHF is a rare occurrence in treated hypertensive subjects.

It is also of interest that the term *"benign essential hypertension"* was still commonly used in the 1950s, largely I believe, because of authoritative statements from experts and in textbooks. The thinking of many physicians at the time seemed to be that not too much could be done to lower blood pressure anyway without significantly changing the patient's quality of life, so a wait and see attitude made some sense—*above all do no harm*. But attitudes about the effectiveness, simplicity, and benefits of therapy were to change dramatically.

The Diuretic Era

Management was greatly simplified in 1958 with the introduction of orally effective diuretics.[25] Difficult cases became easier to manage. The importance of this type of therapy was initially underestimated by some investigators. For example, our group reported that thiazides "were an adjunct to therapy" in subjects who had not been controlled by a ganglion blocking agent, mecamylamine, or other medications.[26] When a thiazide was added to other drugs, blood pressure response was often dramatic (Table III). Normotensive levels were not, however, achieved in some patients with severe hypertension despite the use of triple drug therapy. It soon became apparent to most investigators that many patients with less severe disease actually responded to thiazides as monotherapy. It is of interest to note that chlorothiazide, the first orally effective agent in this group of compounds, was originally studied because of its effectiveness in CHF, not as an antihypertensive agent.

β-Blocking drugs were next on the horizon, presenting more choices with fewer side effects than the other available sympathetic blockers.

Table III. Blood Pressure Response to Chlorothiazide[26]				
	# Cases	Average BP Before Addition of Chlorothiazide*	Average BP After Addition of Chlorothiazide**	Average BP Change
Chlorothiazide	15	174/108	159/100	-15/-8
Rauwolfia (+Chlorothiazide)	39	184/112	166/98	-18/-14
Hydralazine Reserpine (+Chlorothiazide)	17	170/102	156/94	-14/-8
Mecamylamine Hydralazine Reserpine (+Chlorothiazide)	35	174/101	154/85	-20/-16
Total	106			

*Represents blood pressure (BP) after prolonged therapy with drugs other than chlorothiazide
**Average duration of therapy, 7 months

Research Efforts Continued as Therapy Improved

In the 1940s and 1950s research into the causes of hypertension continued as newer therapies were introduced. Dr. Page attempted to explain the mystery of hypertension as a mosaic (Fig. 2).[27] Many of the drugs that were and still are being used affect some of the factors noted in the "mosaic" theory of hypertension.[28] For example, ß-blockers, angiotensin-converting enzyme (ACE) inhibitors or A_{11} receptor antagonists block the effects of the sympathetic nervous system or the renin angiotensin aldosterone system. ß-Blockers reduce the contractile force and rate of the heart beat; diuretics increase excretion of sodium and water; calcium channel blockers (CCBs) block the effects of calcium on smooth muscle and are effective vasodilators, etc. More recently genes

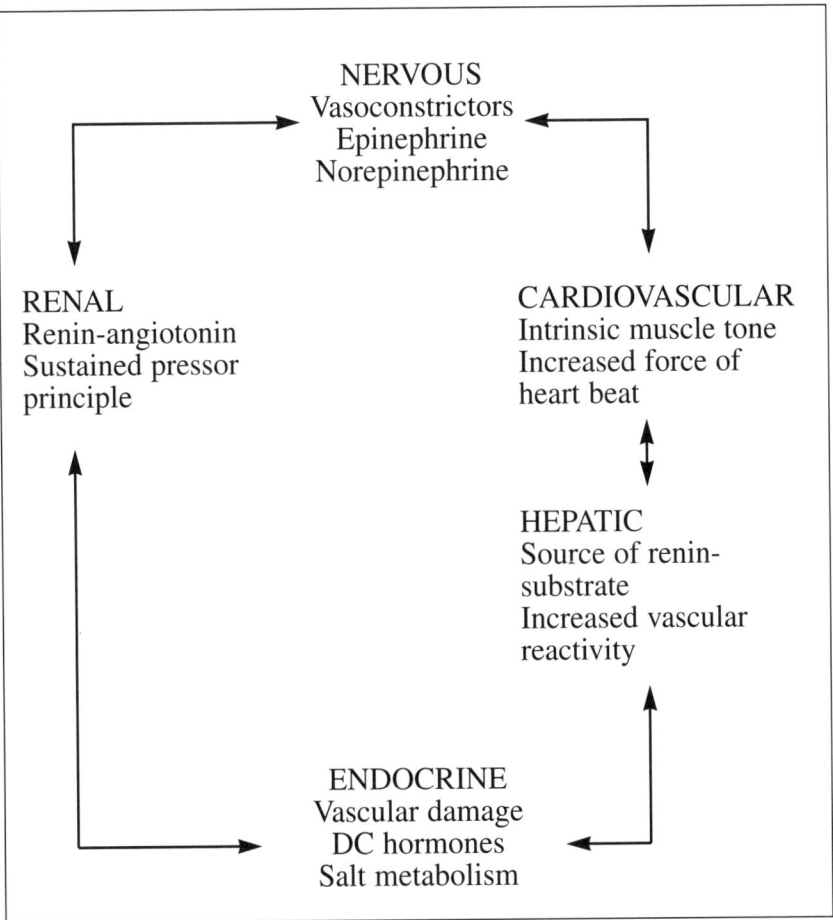

Figure 2. The Page mosaic theory—possible causative factors of hypertension[27] involving neurogenic, renal, hepatic, and endocrine systems.[27]

and gene mutations have been identified that someday may lead to the development of therapies that more specifically address the basic mechanisms that Dr. Page envisioned.

Results of Treatment Improved

As research into mechanisms continued, treatment results improved dramatically. Results can be illustrated by the case of a 29-year-old black woman who was first seen in 1954 with accelerated hypertension, with blood pressures ranging from 220–260/140–160 mm Hg, severe headaches, LVH, and papilledema (Fig. 3). Renal function had deteriorated to only a slight degree with a blood urea nitrogen of 26 mg/dL prior to therapy. She was initially treated with parenteral ganglion blocking agents. Subsequently, many different medications, including an oral ganglion blocking drug (mecamylamine), hydralazine, and guanethidine, were used. She was followed for more than 20 years. Medication was simplified after 1958 and her blood pressure was controlled at normal levels on a rauwolfia–HCTZ combination. Her fundi and electrocardiogram (ECG) normalized, and the blood urea nitrogen remained at between 15 and 18 mg/dL. Prior to the advent of modern therapy, the statistical chances of survival for more than a year for a patient of this severity were less than 5%–10%.

Another example of how the addition of newer medications improved outcome is a 42-year-old man with severe hypertension with LVH and normal kidney function. He was asymptomatic when first seen in 1953 for a routine insurance examination. He was certain that his initial, as well as subsequent blood pressures of 220–260/130–150 mm Hg prior to therapy, were "a mistake." His pressure was only partially controlled from 1953 to 1958, until

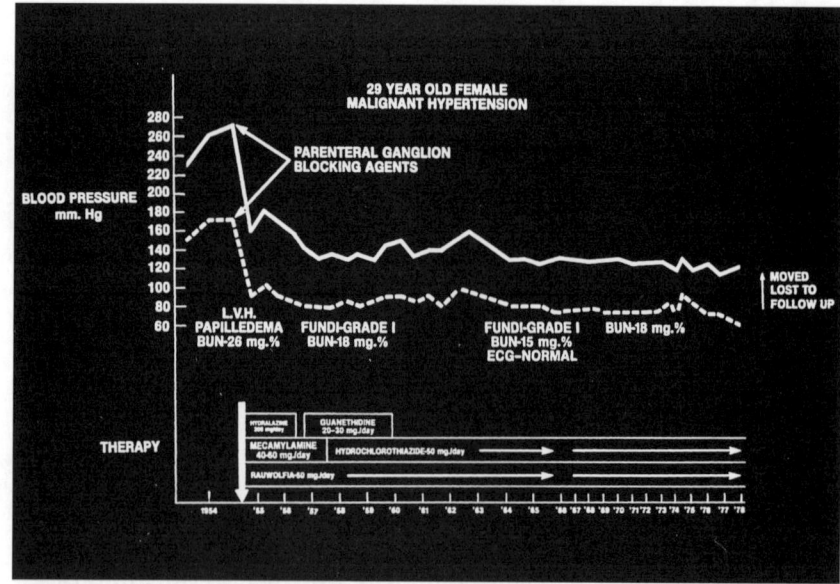

Figure 3. Reversal of "malignant hypertension" by effective blood pressure lowering medications in various combinations. Blood pressures remained within normal limits on hydrochlorothiazide and a rauwolfia preparation from 1966 to 1975 when the patient moved to another state. BUN = blood urea nitrogen; ECG = electrocardiogram

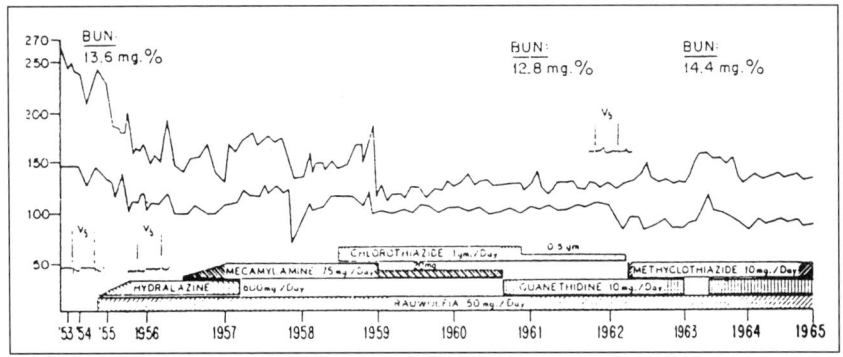

Figure 4. A 42-year-old male with stage IV hypertension and left ventricular hypertrophy. Erratic partial response to rauwolfia, hydralazine, and ganglion blocking agents was noted until 1958–1959 when a thiazide diuretic was added. Patient's blood pressure remained within normal limits from 1965–1978 on a diuretic and β-blocker. He died suddenly at the age of 67 while chopping wood. BUN = blood urea nitrogen

thiazide diuretics were added to his regimen of sympathetic blocking agents, reserpine, and hydralazine. Left ventricular hypertrophy regressed and blood pressure normalized (Fig. 4). Drugs and dosages were changed after 1965 and he lived until 1978. He died at the age of 67 of a ruptured aortic aneurysm, which occurred while he was chopping wood. This patient would probably not have survived for longer than 3–5 years after 1953 without effective antihypertensive drug therapy. While his enjoyment of life was often compromised during his early treatment years, he remained relatively asymptomatic for the last 15–20 years of his life.

Moyer[29] described improvement or slowing down of renal function impairment, even in the prediuretic era, with the antihypertensive medications that were often difficult to manage—ganglion blocking agents, hydralazine, and rauwolfia drugs. For example, in subjects with markedly decreased glomerular filtration rates (40–59 mL/min), only 20% of the treated subjects had expired in 2–5 years compared to a 100% mortality in the untreated group. In subjects with less severe decreases in glomerular filtration rates (80–99 mL/min), 13% of the treated subjects were dead compared to 33% in the untreated group (Table IV). Our experience suggested at that time that, although renal function occasionally decreased initially with an increase in creatinine and blood urea nitrogen as blood pressure was lowered, it most often returned to pretreatment levels after a few weeks and remained there for many years if blood pressure control was maintained.

Table IV. Mortality of Hypertensive Patients Related to Glomerular Filtration Rate: Follow-up 2–5 Years

Initial GFR (mL/min)	# Treated	% Dead Treated	# Untreated	% Dead Untreated
> 100	19	10	14	36
80–99	15	13	9	33
60–79	16	19	12	50
40–59	5	20	10	100
< 40	7	43	9	100
Total	62	18*	54	61†

GFR = glomerular filtration rate
*Number of deaths due to uremia
†15 deaths due to uremia
Decrease in mortality in treated hypertensive subjects with impaired renal function compared to untreated control group
Medications used included hydralazine, rauwolfia drugs, and ganglion blocking agents[29]

Sjoerdsma commented in the journal *Circulation* as late as August 1963 that:

> I look on the work of physicians who pursued
> the drug approach in hypertension as
> being well nigh heroic.

Perhaps it had been, but as the years progressed newer therapies were introduced. We learned to use the older medications more appropriately and treatment was simplified.

Therapeutic Nihilism—An Attitude That Was Difficult to Overcome

But even as results of therapy in the 1950s and early 1960s improved, progress was still held back by prevailing attitudes of therapeutic nihilism, popularized and given respectability by several leading medical authorities.[30] It is hard to believe, but some experts still believed that arterial disease was the cause of hypertension rather than the result. These opinions scoffed at the use of drugs as treatment of the manometer or the "numbers" rather than the patient. There was disbelief that benefit could be achieved by just paying attention to numbers. In the mid 1950s at the New York Academy of Medicine, we presented 10 cases of malignant hypertension, who had experienced clearing of funduscopic abnormalities and heart failure as a result of blood pressure lowering. Two eminent authorities pronounced that this probably represented the "natural history" of some patients. When reversal of LVH was demonstrated on ECG, a well known New York City electrocardiographer sent us a note—"Ain't nature grand"—he expressed disbelief that cardiac hypertrophy could be reversed by just lowering the blood pressure (paying attention to the manometer). In view of more recent data, this attitude seems strange indeed.

But some hypertension experts in the 1990s still belittle the benefits of "just lowering blood pressure." It may be true that modifying other risk factors in addition to lowering blood pressure will result in a greater reduction in morbidity and mortality than has been noted thus far in the clinical trials and clinical experience. But it should be remembered that the major, randomized, placebo-controlled hypertension treatment trials *to date* have only focused on testing the benefit of blood pressure lowering, without specific efforts to lower cholesterol levels, decrease smoking or alcohol intake, or increase exercise. We have good data suggesting that, despite the lack of attempts to reduce other risk factors, the lowering of blood pressure has prevented progression from less severe to more severe disease, reduced the occurrence of LVH and heart failure, and reduced strokes and coronary heart disease (CHD) events in treated compared to control subjects.[31] At present, we have no data to substantiate the belief that the use of newer drugs or attention to factors other than blood pressure will improve outcome to a greater degree than has thus far been accomplished. As noted, it is quite possible that additional benefit will be noted. Hopefully, ongoing studies will answer the question about benefit *beyond just blood pressure lowering*.

Ongoing Concerns About Therapy

In the 1950s and even in the 1960s side effects from therapy were common and the fact that treatment was often complicated and difficult continued to provide excuses not to treat. Data on benefit were being ignored and, for many physicians, anecdotal information from a series of 10 or 20 cases were not enough to convince them to treat even moderately severe hypertensives. They would wait for more data and, perhaps more importantly, therapy that was easier to manage.

In 1965 Pickering, who was one of the pioneers in the study and treatment of hypertension, listed his 3 cautions to be followed in treatment:[32]

1) Never frighten your patient. Many of the symptoms of mild or moderate elevations of pressure are due, not to the hypertension, but to the fear of disease produced directly or indirectly by the doctor.

2) Avoid all unnecessary instrumentation or testing.

3) Avoid petty interference with liberty and the enjoyment of life—*medicine is not yet liberated from the medieval idea that disease is the result of sin and must be expiated by mortification of the flesh.* Patients with elevated arterial pressure should not be allowed to become fat, otherwise restrictions should only be imposed because of the presence of complications and not from fear of them.

Prophetic words for modern day therapists who often 1) frighten patients with the mistaken notion that fear increases adherence to therapy; 2) perform tests that are often expensive and may not result in treatment changes; or 3) still insist on programs or lifestyle changes that they themselves would not be willing to follow.

Patients and physicians continued to be concerned about the side effects of drugs and interference with the enjoyment of life in the treatment of a disease where symptoms were not common. A television program about hypertension in the early 1960s was entitled, "If it only hurt a little." Then we might have been able to convince more patients to accept therapy and more doctors to become involved—in efforts to relieve a patient's symptoms.

A classification of hypertension and a treatment program accepted by most physicians in 1960 are summarized in Tables V and VI. Friedberg in his 1966 edition of *Diseases of the Heart* seemed to agree with these definitions and approaches to management:

> In a patient with *mild benign hypertension,*
> i.e., blood pressure < 220/< 100 mm Hg there
> is no indication for use of hypotensive
> drugs. Continued observation is desirable
> and conservative treatment consisting of
> reassurance, mild sedatives, and weight
> reduction is indicated.[33]

Blood pressure levels up to 220/100 mm Hg were still considered in 1966 to represent "mild benign" hypertension. We were making progress but apparently not among some prominent physi-

Table V. Classification of Hypertension in 1960			
	Grade I (Mild)	Grade II (Moderate)	Grade III (Severe)
BP (mm Hg)	150–200/90–120	180–250/110–150	190–250/120–160
Symptoms	Few or none	May have early morning headaches but generally feels well	Some retinal changes, possible hemorrhages
Changes in heart or retina	Few—detectable by routine exam	Some arteriolar narrowing or nicking; some slight heart enlargement	Heart enlargement
Urine	Negative	Usually normal or trace of albumin	Albumin
Kidney function	Normal		
Five-year mortality without specific treatment	30%	45%	80%
BP = blood pressure			

Table VI. Treatment of Hypertension—1960				
Classification	Initial Treatment	Subsequent Treatment	Next Step	Next Step
Grade I	None in most cases; mild sedative; 2–4 g salt diet; 250 mg chlorothiazide	Add 0.15 g phenobarbital 2–3 x daily	Add reserpine 0.25 mg bid	Hydralazine Hexamethonium Pentolinium Chlorison-domine Tartrate Mecamylamine
Grade II	Low-sodium diet with chlorothiazide bid plus reserpine 0.25 mg bid; in many patients hydralazine or a ganglion blocker			

cians. Friedberg also noted that:

> "a psychopathologic personality is said to be associated with hypertension."

> "many of the symptoms of patients with hypertension are regarded as psychoneurotic"

> "sedatives, barbiturates, bromides, meprobomate, and chloral hydrate are the drugs most commonly used in hypertensive patients"[33]—although these may not be effective in cases of "fixed" hypertension.

These statements were reminiscent of a widely distributed ad from the Metropolitan Life Insurance Company which appeared in magazines such as National Geographic in 1957:

Doctors are trying to learn more about high blood pressure or hypertension which affects an estimated 6 million Americans.

"Fortunately hypertension can often be controlled simply by reducing day to day emotional stresses which push blood pressure up and tend to keep it excessively elevated."

Even a major life insurance company that had helped to clarify the risks of elevated blood pressure had not recognized that stress was not a major cause of hypertension and that stress reduction was not a definitive treatment—and they failed to recognize that many more than 6 million Americans had blood pressures high enough to increase thier risk of CV disease—primarily because the levels of blood pressure considered to be hypertensive at that time were considerably higher that 140/90 mm Hg.

The use of the thiazides in "mild" hypertension was, however, being recommended by some physicians; the use of other agents was now being suggested in more severe cases.

It happened that many of the "doubters," like Goldring, Chasis, and Perrera, were found in New York City—Midwesterners, like Page, Dustan, Perry, Schroeder, and Gifford, and Wilkins and Freis, investigators from Boston and Washington, had accepted data that treatment was beneficial and were pursuing it vigorously.

We had certainly progressed from 1950 when psychosurgery (resection of portions of the frontal lobe) was used by some to reduce stress and lower blood pressure. This procedure was carried out in desperation and as a corollary of the psychosomatic theories of essential hypertension. Data were meager, but some investigators reported a lowering of blood pressure and symptomatic improvement.[34]

The Clinical Trials—1960s–1980s

From the 1960s to the early 1980s several major clinical studies established the fact that early treatment of hypertension would prevent complications and prolong life. These studies have been extensively reviewed elsewhere, but a short summary is appropriate. The Veterans Administration Study[35] was a controlled study on a group of male patients with moderately severe and severe hypertension (diastolic blood pressures as high as 125–130 mm Hg). A lowering of blood pressure with medication dramatically improved prognosis in treated compared to placebo subjects (medications used included diuretics, reserpine, hydralazine, etc.). Acute pulmonary edema and heart failure were virtually eliminated and the number of strokes, both hemorrhagic and thrombotic, was markedly decreased. A statistically significant decrease in the incidence of myocardial infarction or death from coronary artery disease was not, however, documented in treated patients over a short period of time, although there was a trend in that direction. In the cohort of subjects with less severe disease, similar findings were noted.

The U.S. Public Health Study on Mild Hypertension[36] confirmed the findings of the Veterans Administration Study in less severe subjects—"hypertensive" complications were reduced and progression to more severe disease prevented—but no proof was forthcoming that the mortality from myocardial infarction or sudden death was reduced by therapy—again a trend in that direction was noted. It was not unexpected that a statistically significant difference failed to be achieved in this study of a relatively small number of young men with less severe hypertension where the incidence of coronary disease was low and differences between treated and untreated groups difficult to establish. Table VII summarizes the morbidity and mortality results in patients with stages I and II hypertension in 5 of the early hypertension treatment trials. These pooled results indicate a reduction in morbidity and mortality in treated compared to control subjects.

The Hypertension, Detection and Follow-Up Program Study (HDFP)[37] attempted to clarify the effects of blood pressure lowering on less severe degrees of hypertension. This was a multicenter study involving approximately 11,000 men and women that, although its design has been faulted, answered several questions. In this study, more than 5,000 patients underwent rigorous treatment to achieve goal blood pressure levels, utilizing a stepped-care (SC) method of therapy. This was similar to a program outlined in the 1977 JNC (diuretics as first-step therapy, reserpine or, later in the study, propranolol, as second-step therapy, and hydralazine as third-step therapy).[38] Another group of 5,000 patients were returned to their communities for usual and customary care which, in many cases, also included antihypertensive drug therapy. At the end of 5 years, systolic and diastolic blood pressures had been reduced in both groups but to a lower level in the vigorously treated group (a difference of -12/-5 mm Hg in the SC treated compared to the referred-care group). Blood pressure had been reduced to goal in a higher percentage of SC treated than less vigorously treated patients (65% vs. 45%). Overall mortality was reduced to a greater degree in the specially treated group, with a 45% reduction in

Table VII. Treatment Trials of Stage I and II Hypertension: Fatal and Nonfatal Cardiac and Cerebrovascular Events in Control and Treated Groups*

Complications	Control		Treated		
	#**	%	#**	%	% Improvement
Total morbid events	563	9.0	417	6.6	27
Total mortality	342	5.4	252	4.1	24
Cerebrovascular events: fatal & nonfatal	140	2.2	76	1.2	50
Fatal coronary events	79	1.2	46	0.7	42

*Data from a subset of patients in the Veterans Administration Cooperative Study, United States Public Health Cooperative Study, Hypertension Detection and Follow-up Program: stratum I, Australian Study, and Oslo Study
**Total control and treated populations each comprise approximately 6,400 subjects

stroke mortality rates and, importantly, a reduction of 20% in deaths from myocardial infarction, when compared with the less vigorously treated patients. Benefit was noted, in each of the groups with less severe hypertension, i.e., diastolic pressures of 90–94, 95–99 and 100–104 mm Hg. Of great importance was the fact that, although mortality and morbidity were reduced even in those patients who were treated *after* the onset of target-organ involvement (target organ damage [TOD]), the level from which risk was reduced was considerably higher—a strong argument for early treatment before evidence of complications (Table VIII), i.e., mortality was reduced equally by 22% in subjects with and without TOD, but mortality rate in SC and referred-care was considerably higher in patients with TOD than in subjects without TOD (15.6 compared to 4.5 and 20 compared to 5.8).

Table VIII. Hypertension Detection and Follow-up Program: Percentage Reduction in Mortality in Stratum-1 Subjects (Diastolic Blood Pressure 90–104 mm Hg) According to Presence or Absence of Pretreatment Target-Organ Damage[37]

Entry Characteristics	Stepped-Care			Referred-Care			
	Sample Size	# Deaths	Mortality Rate	Sample Size	# Deaths	Mortality Rate	Reduction in Mortality
Target-organ damage present*	501	78	**15.6**	460	92	**20.0**	**22.0**
Target-organ damage absent	3,402	153	**4.5**	3,462	199	**5.8**	**22.4**

*Target-organ damage included left ventricular hypertrophy on the electrocardiogram, history of myocardial infarction, stroke, intermittent claudication, or a serum creatinine greater than 1.7 mg/dL

The HDFP study has been criticized because of the lack of a placebo group, but benefits in this study were probably underestimated as a result of the study design. If the group on less rigorous therapy (the control or usual care group) had not been treated at all, blood pressure differences would have been greater and benefit most probably would also have been greater. The HDFP data had important implications for treatment recommendations in subsequent JNC reports. Many of the hypertension experts in the U.S. concurred with the results and suggested treatment of patients with persistent diastolic pressures above 90 mm Hg, with or without evidence of TOD, but some still did not.

Despite data from the HDFP and other studies, the concept persisted that little benefit resulted from treating mild or less severe hypertension. Part of the problem related to recurrent claims that a reduction in CHD events had not been demonstrated in several of the trials. It is important to note that studies such as the Australian trial[39] or the first Medical Research Council study[40] were not designed to test this hypothesis and lacked the power to do so. Too few CHD events occurred in the placebo or control groups in these trials for a meaningful comparison to be made. For example, in the Australian trial, less than 50% of the predicted CHD events occurred in the placebo group—with so few events, it was difficult to demonstrate benefit of treatment. But, as noted in Table V, when data from the Veterans Administration Cooperative Study in less severe hypertension, the U.S. Public Health Cooperative Study, the HDFP stratum I (less severe hypertensives), the Australian, and the Oslo studies were combined, total mortality was reduced by 24% and fatal coronary events by 42% in treated, compared to control or placebo subjects. Despite these facts, many physicians continued to make the claim that benefit of treatment of less severe hypertension had not been demonstrated.

The Question of Drug Dosages

In the 1960s we were still using medications that caused numerous side effects or adverse reactions—centrally acting drugs such as methyldopa and clonidine, monoamine oxidase inhibitors, vasodilators such as hydralazine, and potent sympathetic blockers. *Dosages were higher than necessary.* We had not realized that dose response curves for these agents were not often linear—that 300 mg/day of hydralazine was not always more effective than 150 mg or that 600 mg would necessarily lower blood pressure more than 300 mg. Yet some investigators were using doses as high as 1 g or more a day—positive antinuclear antibody tests were common and cases of lupus were reported at these higher dosages[16]—discouraging findings for physicians who had any doubts about treatment benefits. Physicians in the U.K. were using propranolol in dosages up to 3 g a day—subsequent observations determined that most of the patients who respond to propranolol will respond to doses of 80–240 mg/day, with fewer adverse reactions. Small wonder that patients were fatigued or impotent and that many physicians were reluctant to use any medications to treat people with less severe disease. We have since learned that with many drugs, including the diuretics, ACE inhibitors, ß-blockers, etc., the percentage of responders does not always increase as dosage increases. Smaller doses often produce almost as great an effect as larger ones.[41]

Major problems were created as a result of this "the more the better" approach. When 1.0 or more mg/day of reserpine was given, a serious depression occurred in some patients. (It was subsequently established that an effective dosage with few side effects is about 0.05–0.10 mg/day).[42] Central inhibitors such as α-methyldopa caused fatigue and depression in large doses (2–3 g/day); 250–750 mg will often produce almost identical decreases in blood pressure with fewer side effects. The use of guanethidine resulted in syncope if the dosage was not carefully controlled. It was also established that a majority of responders to diuretics did so at doses of 25–50 mg or the equivalent of HCTZ (using 100–200 mg/day increased the percentage of responders to some degree but also increased adverse reactions). Dosage response was usually not linear; most antihypertensive drugs produced most of their desirable effects at lower doses, and if these proved ineffective, small doses of another class of drug could be added with better results than using larger doses of one agent.[41,43]

An example of the use of multiple drugs in small doses was SER-AP-ES, which was marketed as a diuretic-antihypertensive combination containing 3 compounds: 1) reserpine (0.1 mg), described as "a mild antihypertensive with a calming and heart-slowing action;" 2) hydralazine hydrochloride (25 mg), whose action was summarized as "a potent antihypertensive which increases renal circulation and relaxes cerebral vascular tone;" and 3) HCTZ (15 mg), with antihypertensive and potent diuretic effects. The average maintenance dosage was about 1 tablet taken 2–3 times a day. At that time the regimen was considered easy to follow and simple for the busy physician to implement, although the 3 times a day dosage was often a problem.

In 1970 SER-AP-ES was the leading drug used in the treatment of hypertension, with more than 38,000 physicians prescribing it and with sales of over 16 million dollars annually. It is of interest to compare these numbers with 1996 statistics—several of the leading antihypertensive medications each have sales in excess of 1 billion dollars annually.

Physicians apparently accepted the concept of fixed dosage combination therapy in the late 1960s and 1970s because results of treatment were quite satisfactory.

The Dilemma of "Mild Hypertension"

In 1978 Dr. William McFate Smith, using Hamlet's soliloquy, expressed the ongoing dilemma of treating patients with less severe hypertension who were relatively asymptomatic[44] and poetically described the problems with available therapy:

> *TO TREAT OR NOT TO TREAT*
> With apologies to the Bard
>
> To treat, or not to treat: that is the question.
> Whether tis nobler in the mind to suffer
> The risks and complications of hypertension,
> Or to take a potion against these ravages,
> And by opposing end them? To awake; to live;
> For sure; and by some drugs to say we end
> The strokes and heart attacks
> That flesh is heir to, tis a consummation
> Devoutly to be wished.
>
> To awake; to live;
> To live? perchance to love. Ah there's the rub;
> For in that living, and loving, what fate may come
> When we take our pills, must give us pause.
> There's the impotence that makes calamity

of a long life;
For who would bear the whips and scorns of that;
The limp response, the lover's pity,
The pangs of lost esteem, the end of "macho";
The insensitivity of healers and the spurns
That the patient suffers when he himself
Might his therapy adjust?

Who would these afflictions bear,
This dysfunction and depression,
But that the dread of disability and death,
Whose consequences are so certain
 and so hopeless
That we rather take those pills we have
Than fly to others we know not of:
Or not at all.

Thus, conscience doth make cowards of us all;
And thus the certain risk of hypertension,
Is sicklied o'er with the pale cast of doubt,
That benefit exceeds the risk and inconvenience,
And trials of great cost and moment
Must be mounted,
Or miss the time for action.

More clinical trials were mounted—we did not miss the time for action.

The Newer Drugs—and New Major Trials

In the 1970s and 1980s the information that hypertension was an important risk factor for heart and vascular disease and that effective and acceptable treatment was finally available was being widely disseminated. The NHBPEP helped to inform the public that strokes and heart attacks could be prevented by the effective treatment of hypertension and that while reassurance, sedation, weight loss, and sodium restriction might be helpful in some patients, it was not definitive therapy in the majority. But more data were needed to convince more physicians and patients that the effort, possible inconvenience and cost of therapy in less severe cases were worth it. Large clinical trials were undertaken to confirm, if possible, the benefits of therapy in less severe cases of hypertension and in the elderly, a rapidly growing segment of the population with a high prevalence of hypertension and a high incidence of complications attributable to elevated blood pressure. The pharmaceutical industry had been actively searching for more effective and better tolerated medications— and they found them. Nonpharmacologic approaches to therapy continued to be a part of the treatment regimen, but it was recognized that advances in pharmacologic therapy had made a major difference in outcome.

The availability of α-blockers, α-ß-blockers, converting enzyme inhibitors, and CCBs in the 1970s and 1980s increased choices and made therapy easier to carry out in many patients. Response rates were increased and side effects reduced by utilizing combinations of small doses of different classes of drugs. No longer were we punishing people "for the sin of having high blood pressure." We were lowering blood pressure without major side effects in most, although not all, cases.[45] The benefit/risk ratio of treating the less severe and relatively asymptomatic hypertensive patient had increased considerably.

The Reports of the Joint National Committees on Detection, Evaluation and Treatment of High Blood Pressure

The JNC Reports were first issued in 1977.[38] The NHLBI had appointed a committee composed of representatives from most of the major medical organizations. The committee formulated suggestions for the routine evaluation and treatment of hypertension. Since that time these committees have been convened approximately every 4 years and continue to issue guidelines for treatment. The initial guidelines for follow-up observation were conservative but did suggest that if the diastolic blood pressure was greater than 120 mm Hg, prompt evaluation was called for. If blood pressures were higher than 160/95 mm Hg in a person less than 50 years of age, they were to be checked in a month, *but over the age of 50 not too much attention was to be paid to this less severe degree of hypertension* (we had little data on benefits of lowering blood pressure in the elderly and many investigators still did not consider hypertension a serious problem in this age group). In fact, the British literature in 1974–1978 was advising physicians that:

> Antihypertensive agents produce no obvious benefit in patients over 65.

Fry J., Lancet. 1974

> Diastolic blood pressures of up to 120 mm Hg in symptomless elderly hypertensives are not an indication for therapy.

Kennedy R.D., Modern Geriatrics. 1974

and

> Hypotensive drugs should probably not be given (in the elderly) unless the blood pressure is more than 200/110 mm Hg.

Editorial, Br Med J. 1978

While definitive data on benefit of therapy were not yet available in this group of patients, this was long after data from epidemiologic studies had confirmed that increasing blood pressures in the elderly increased the risk of cardiovascular disease.

Over the years, as more information became available, the committee recommended more careful follow-up and more vigorous therapy at lower levels of pressure. The JNC V, published in 1993, changed definitions of hypertension to highlight the importance of systolic blood pressure as a major risk factor for heart disease.[46] It became important to get rid of the long-standing statement that a systolic blood pressure of 100 plus a person's age was "normal." Persistent blood pressures > 140/90 mm Hg in the young *and* the elderly were now considered indications for treatment—initially, lifestyle modifications, but if these proved ineffective, pharmacologic therapy. Data from many long-term clinical trials in the 1970s–1990s had established the science to justify this approach to therapy.[37,39,40,47–50] Lowering of blood pressure with antihypertensive agents had been shown to reduce morbidity and mortality in middle-aged *and* older individuals; benefit clearly outweighed the risk and possible inconvenience of therapy, even in less severe cases.[51]

Worldwide Recommendations Differ

The recent 1996 report of the World Health Organization suggests that individuals with elevated blood pressure levels of 140–160/90–95 mm Hg, *without* evidence of "target organ damage (TOD)" should be "followed." Drug therapy should be used in subjects with blood pressures ≥ 160/≥ 95 mm Hg even if there is no evidence of TOD, but only those with a high cardiovascular risk (TOD) should be treated with medication if blood pressures are higher than 140/90 mm Hg but below 160/95 mm Hg. Many experts disagree with this approach and agree with the JNC V recommendation—a persistent blood pressure of > 140/90 mm Hg, with or *without* TOD or significant other cardiovascular risk factors, should be treated. A strong argument can be made, based on our present knowledge, that if blood pressure can be lowered in individuals with less severe hypertension, before evidence of TOD, and if this can be achieved without interfering with the enjoyment of life, and with relatively little cost, then it represents a reasonable approach to management. Although the absolute risk to a patient with this degree of disease is not great, even this low risk can probably be reduced. From a public health point of view, this approach also makes sense. Since a large majority of hypertensive patients have "less severe" (stage I or II) hypertension, reducing disability in this group will have a major impact on the cost of care and the quality of life of many millions of people.

Pharmacoeconomists, however, might agree with the WHO recommendations and emphasize the point that the most "cost effective" approach to treatment is to treat older persons or persons with at least 1–2 risk factors for cardiovascular disease in addtion to hypertension. Here, the benefits of treatment are more immediate and dramatic—the higher the risk, the greater the benefit—at least over the short term of the clinical trials. It may take longer to detect a mortality-morbidity decrease in low risk individuals. We may never have adequate 10–15 year follow up data on treatment results since trialsof this length may never be done. "Soft" data from the MRFIT and HDFP studies at 10.5 and 8.3 years suggest that benefit, i.e., reduction of CHD events, does increase over time.

Stepped-Care (SC)

The SC regimen elaborated in the JNC Report in 1977 suggested thiazide diuretics as initial therapy with reserpine, methyldopa, or propranolol (which wasn't yet approved for treatment of hypertension) to be given if blood pressure was not controlled by nonpharmacologic means. Hydralazine, guanethidine, or clonidine could be added if necessary to reduce pressure to goal levels (Table IX).

As noted, this report reflected a lack of emphasis on treatment of the older age groups. The 1980,[52] 1984,[53] and 1988[54] reports recognized that risk in the elderly was clearly defined and that there was benefit to treatment. The JNC V in 1993 reviewed all of the major randomized studies in the elderly from the late 1980s that had demonstrated a marked decrease in strokes, CHD events, CHF, and all cardiovascular events in treated, compared to control or placebo patients and, as noted, recommended lowering blood pressure to goal levels of below 140/90 mm Hg if at all possible, in all ages.

In 1980 the JNC recommended thiazide diuretics and ß-blockers as initial therapy.[52] If blood pressure control was not achieved, clonidine, guanabenz, reserpine, or methyldopa were suggested as possible step 2 drugs (Table IX). If one of these combinations proved ineffective, it was suggested that a vasodilator such as hydralazine or minoxidil be added. If patients still had not responded to goal blood pressures of < 140/90 mm Hg, the use of quanethidine was suggested. This agent is potent and its use often converted a resistant patient to one with normotensive blood pressure levels. But titration of dosage was difficult and side effects such as dizziness, syncope, etc., were not uncommon. Other agents such as methyldopa and clonidine were suggested in 1980 and in 1984 (Table IX) as alternative therapies. These agents are not used extensively today and have been replaced by ACE inhibitors or CCBs that are better tolerated.

Controversies About Stepped-Care

There has been a great deal of controversy about the stepped-care approach to therapy, i.e., the concept that if drug A doesn't work, add drug B in small doses, etc. Dr. Page, in an editorial in *Modern Medicine*, in 1985, put the debate in perspective:

> We must not get snarled in nonproblems
> such as whether stepped-care is good or

Table IX. Evolution of the Recommendations of the Joint National Committees on Detection Evaluation and Treatment of High Blood Pressure (JNC)*

JNC I (1977) Stepped-Care	JNC II (1980) Stepped-Care	JNC III (1984) Stepped-Care	JNC IV (1988) Individualized Stepped-Care	JNC V (1993) Modified Stepped-Care
1. Diuretics	1. Diuretics	1. Less than full dose of diuretic or β-blocker	1. Diuretic, β-blocker, calcium antagonist, or ACE inhibitor	1. Diuretic or β-blocker. Alternative therapy: ACE inhibitor, CCB, α-β-blocker, or α₁-blocker
2. Add methyldopa, reserpine, or propranolol	2. Adrenergic inhibiting agents—clonidine, methyldopa, β-blocking drugs, α₁-blocker, rauwolfia	2. Add small dose of adrenergic inhibiting agent or thiazide-type diuretic	2. Add second drug of different class; increase dose of first drug or substitute a drug of a different class**	2. Increase dose or substitute another drug, or add a second agent from a different class**
3. Add hydralazine or clonidine	3. Hydralazine	3. Add a vasodilator	3. Add third drug of a different class** or substitute second drug	3. Add a second or third agent and/or diuretic if not already prescribed
4. Add or substitute guanethidine	4. Guanethidine	4. Add guanethidine	4. Add third or fourth drug**	

*All 5 JNCs had recommended nonpharmacologic therapy prior to the use of medication

**Classes of drugs: diuretics, β-blockers, calcium antagonists, angiotensin-converting enzyme (ACE) inhibitors, α$_{II}$ receptor antagonists, α₁-blockers, centrally acting α₂ agonist, rauwolfia drugs, α-β blockers, and vasodilators

bad. Stepped-care is merely a way of
orderly thinking: an attempt to present
an orderly scenario in what otherwise
threatens to join the New Yorkers
Department of Utter Confusion.

The algorithms for treatment presented by the JNCs were suggestions—they were not appropriate for everyone, but they proved
to be helpful to busy practitioners who did not have time to investi-
gate the nuances of care. They represented the opinions of experts
and a summary of evidence on benefit. The SC approach allows a
great deal of individualization and has been successful in a majority
of cases. The attack on the concept of SC was probably based more
on promotional efforts to encourage physicians to change prescribing patterns away from the use of the medications that had been
used in the trials, most specifically, diuretics and ß-blockers, than it
was on treatment results or science.

Myths and Facts

Frequently in clinical medicine (and in other areas as well), speculations, hypotheses, or theories are presented as fact without adequate scientific data to support them. If these are widely disseminated and repeated often enough, especially by persons of authori-
ty, it becomes more and more difficult to distinguish fact from
fancy. Nowhere is this better illustrated than in the efforts to
change prescribing habits of physicians in the late 1970s, the mid
1980s, and early 1990s when short-term study results were often
extrapolated into long-term speculations, where theories were
often introduced into clinical practice before any data on outcome
of treatment were available, and where promotional activity would
often omit or overemphasize specific data to prove a point. Often
times preliminary data from animal studies were extrapolated to
indicate benefit in humans. These were repeated often and disseminated widely. Many physicians began to accept them as fact
and changed their treatment practices. Over time, however, these
misinterpretations and speculations have gradually been refuted
by evidence from long-term trials and clinical experience.

The latter day (1970s–1990s) myths were no longer based on
lack of knowledge about the risks of hypertension or whether or

not vascular disease caused high blood pressure or vice versa, etc., they were now about specific aspects of therapy which had important economic and treatment ramifications.

Myth. Diuretics increase lipid levels. This partially true observation suggested that if cholesterol and low density lipoprotein (LDL) levels were increased by diuretics, this might help to explain why there has not been a major reduction of CHD events in the clinical trials.

Fact. Increases of 5%–7% in serum cholesterol levels do occur in short-term trials (6 weeks to 1 year) following the use of diuretics, *but* these changes are not noted in trials of longer than 1 year in duration. A review of these trials indicated that cholesterol levels had not increased.[55] Two studies have reported a prolonged elevation of cholesterol levels. Neither reported changes that were statistically significant—one 2-year study included 10 subjects; in the other, 33 subjects entered the study but only 7 remained to be evaluated at the end of 42 months.[56,57] (This latter study was cited 27 times in the medical literature in the 4 years following its publication).

Coronary heart disease events were reduced by a statistically significant degree (16%) in the clinical trials that were diuretic-based.[51] Despite these data the literature continues to include statements that CHD events have not been significantly reduced.

Myth. Patients with hyperlipidemia, especially those with ischemic heart disease, should not be given diuretics or ß-blockers.

Fact. Data do not support this—in several long-term trials, specifically the Systolic Hypertension in the Elderly Program (SHEP)[47] and the HDFP[37] trials that utilized diuretics as initial therapy, patients with hyperlipidemia experienced a similar decrease in cardiovascular events as those subjects with normal lipid levels. In addition, a reduction in CHD morbidity and mortality has been noted with ß-blockers in patients with heart disease, despite their possible adverse effects on triglycerides and high density lipoprotein (HDL) cholesterol levels.

Myth. Calcium channel blockers possess a unique vascular protective activity and are cardioprotective.

Fact. Not proven as yet—this has been demonstrated in animal experiments but may not be true in humans. Thus far, data from several trials in patients with unstable angina or other evidence of ischemic heart disease have failed to demonstrate that CCBs reduce mortality. A reduction in the reinfarction rate by about 20% has been reported with the nondihydropyridine CCBs, i.e., diltiazem and verapamil. The shorter acting dihydropyridines, which may increase heart rate, have not been shown to have a beneficial effect on CHD events and may even be harmful. At present, ß-blockers should probably remain the drugs of choce in postmyocardial infarction patients or subjects with angina unless there are contraindications to their use. CCBs do lower blood pressure and are generally well tolerated. Whether or not additional studies with longer acting formulations of these agents will result in better long term outcome than with other agents in hypertensive subjects remains to be seen. A recent nonrandomized study with a long acting dihydropyridine reported a reduction in strokes and severe arrhythmias. Coronary heart disease morbidity and mortality were not reduced—there were few events in both groups.[83] The argument that the use of CCBs offers more than just a blood pressure lowering effect and that these agents are superior to other medications probably accounts for at least some of the reasons for their widespread use in hypertension, but thus far this speculation remains unproven.

Myth. Quality of life is improved by ACE inhibitors more than with other antihypertensive agents.

Fact. May not be true—numerous studies have reported that quality of life is improved with almost all of the antihypertensive drugs presently being used in relatively small doses, except for the centrally acting agents that were originally compared to an ACE inhibitor. Two recent studies, which compared 6 different classes of drugs with placebo control actually reported the greatest improvement in quality of life measurements with diuretics and ß-blockers.[58,59] Angiotensin-converting enzyme inhibitors are well tolerated by most patients, but this should not be a major reason for specifically choosing this class of medication over another.

Myth. Reduction of sodium, loss of weight, or maintenance of ideal weight, reduction of alcohol intake, and moderate exercise may be all that is necessary to effectively treat hypertension.

Fact. This is a confusing and incorrect message for the public. Although there are some patients who will respond to this type of nonpharmacologic regimen or lifestyle modification approach to therapy, it has been estimated that as many as 75% of patients will not respond and specific antihypertensive therapy will be necessary. Recent clinical trials have reported a decrease in blood pressure of about 8–11/5–7 mm Hg on nonpharmacologic interventions. This is clearly enough to reduce blood pressure to normotensive levels in the patient with less severe hypertension, but many patients in a real world situation are unable to remain on the type of program that clinical trial subjects adhere to. Thus, the majority of patients are not able to achieve this degree of blood pressure lowering. The message should be, as it is in JNC V, that *lifestyle modifications should be tried first* and be continued if they are effective, but if pressures remain above 140/90 mm Hg, specific antihypertensive drug therapy should be employed, *in addition* to nonpharmacologic interventions. In a placebo controlled study comparing various antihypertensive drugs and nutritional intervention, medications reduced blood pressure -7 to -8 /-4 to -5 mm Hg more than lifestyle changes in a group of subjects with less severe hypertension. Overall, cardiovascular events were reduced by almost 50% in the medically treated compared to the lifestyle only groups over a four-year period.[58]

Further Efforts to Change Treatment Practices
As expected, attempts to change treatment practices focused on efforts to wean physicians away from the use of diuretics, since these had been designated as initial therapy in all of the JNC reports and had been used as initial therapy in all of the clinical trials—and were widely used in the 1960s–1980s with good results.

Myth.

> "The adverse effects of diuretics on uric acid metabolism, serum potassium, plasma cholesterol and triglycerides may contribute to *increases* in the incidence of coronary heart disease, angina pectoris, myocardial infarction and congestive heart failure"[60]

This was published in a peer-review journal in 1986 and reflects some prevailing opinions even at this stage in the history of hypertension treatment. Diuretics are described as dangerous drugs, despite the fact that in all of the major diuretic-based clinical trials a reduction, not an increase, in cardiovascular events had been demonstrated.

McInnes, et al[61] answered most of these statements in an article entitled, *Cardiotoxicity and Diuretics, Much Speculation, Little Substance.*

The facts were 1) there was no evidence that the use of diuretics increased angina pectoris—quite the opposite; and that 2) diuretics were routinely used to treat CHF—there was no evidence that they worsened it. Part of this provocative statement, however, is true—uric acid levels may be increased and, at least with high-dose diuretics, potassium levels may be decreased—but the extrapolation of these effects to adverse clinical outcomes were not based on data. One could speculate that they might have been prompted by an effort to induce physicians to change treatment practices.

Additional provocative statements followed in 1989:

> "Diuretics elevate blood sugar, cause overt diabetes, induce diabetic ketoacidosis, elevate total cholesterol and LDL-C, and reduce HDL-C, cause deterioration of renal function and worsening of left ventricular hypertrophy. They are contraindicated in patients with hyperglycemia, hyperlipidemia and coronary heart disease."[62]

Another strong statement that goes beyond the issue of lipid abnormalities and diuretics. This was published in 1989 in a peer-review journal and flies in the face of the available scientific data. Unfortunately, this statement was widely quoted in the medical literature, was cited 54 times in the 3 years after its publication, and discussed at numerous medical meetings. Undoubtedly it influenced many physicians to abandon the use of these relatively inexpensive and highly effective antihypertensive agents. Several review papers and additional studies have carefully documented answers to these exaggerated and misleading statements.[63,64]

Fact. Three- to five-year studies continued to report that morbidity and mortality were reduced, not increased, when diuretics were used. Data continued to contradict the misconception that cholesterol and LDL levels were increased; there was no evidence of an adverse effect on HDL levels. As noted, subsequent outcome data in both the SHEP[47] and the HDFP[37] studies demonstrated the same degree of decrease in morbidity and mortality in patients with elevated cholesterol levels as in those with normal or low cholesterol levels. In addition, although both diuretics and ß-blockers may adversely affect insulin resistance, this action does not appear to have a major effect on outcome. A significant increase in the occurrence of diabetes had not been demonstrated in the 3–5 year trials when diuretics or ß-blockers were used as initial therapy or in combination.[64] A recent follow-up report from the SHEP study[65] noted a greater reduction in cardiovascular morbidity and mortality in diabetics than in non-diabetes in a diuretic-based treatment program. These findings were similar to previous data from the HDFP study.

One case control study has reported no difference in the occurrence of diabetes in hypertensive individuals treated with diuretics compared to ACE inhibitors, CCBs, or ß-blockers.[66] Another retrospective, nonrandomized case control study in insulin-dependent diabetics with severe retinopathy, did however, report that the use of diuretics increased CHD mortality.[67] No data on ongoing therapy or achieved blood pressures were available in this latter report. These data have not been confirmed. *Data from these non-controlled, retrospective analyses may be accepted as hypotheses but should not be relied on for definitive treatment decisions.*

Misconceptions, Speculations, or Misinterpretations of Data and Their Effect on Treatment Practices

NEW STUDY SAYS DIURETICS RAISE HEART ATTACK RISKS*

Diuretics, the most widely used
class of drugs against high
blood pressure, can cause biochemical
changes that make people

more susceptible to heart attacks,
researchers have found...

*N.Y. Times 4/28/89

This provocative headline followed a report that suggested an increase in serum glucose levels and insulin resistance in a four-month comparative study of an ACE inhibitor and a diuretic.[68] The authors presented no data on heart attacks or death and merely hinted that these metabolic changes might be of importance. The effect of the *New York Times* article and national T.V. coverage on physicians and patients who were prescribing and taking diuretics was, as expected, quite dramatic.

A question must be posed: Why have some of these speculations been so widely disseminated? One might assume that, unlike the misconceptions of years ago, many of these more recent pronouncements were elaborated upon as part of promotional activities and not as "misinterpretations" of scientific data. The media, always ready for a sensational story, certainly didn't help. Unfortunately, these examples of misconceptions or extrapolations of data from either short-term or poorly conceived studies have had an influence on approaches to therapy—the use of diuretics and ß-blockers has decreased steadily in the past 10–15 years. It is only within the past year or so that physicians are again beginning to increase their use of diuretics as initial therapy in smaller doses or in combination with ß-blockers, ACE inhibitors, or calcium channel blockers. It is perhaps the realization that the utilization of smaller doses of diuretics may have almost the same effect on blood pressure as large doses that has finally convinced some physicians to begin using them again; or at least to dismiss a great deal of the advertised potential hazards and pay attention to outcome data from the long-term trials. Many of these trial results were achieved, however, with fairly high doses of diuretics.

The rauwolfia drugs had also suffered from the widespread dissemination of anecdotal data—some of which were based on fact, but greatly exaggerated. The use of these agents decreased rapidly in the 1960s and 1970s. Today rauwolfia drugs are rarely prescribed in the U.S. As noted before, in smaller doses, these agents, along with small doses of a diuretic, are highly effective with few major side effects.

Hypokalemia—Sudden Death and Diuretics: Fact or Myth?

Finally, we must address the issue of a reported increase in sudden death when diuretics are given.

Data from the Multiple Risk Factor Intervention Trial (MRFIT)[69,70] had suggested that patients with electrocardiographic abnormalities, who received high doses of diuretics, were at greater risk for sudden death than those who received lower doses, presumably because of hypokalemia. This conclusion, however, represents another example of the misinterpretation of data—a misinterpretation that had an important effect on treatment practices.[71] Careful analyses of the MRFIT study found no significant correlation between the incidence of death and dosages of diuretics and little correlation between the incidence of death and potassium levels measured prior to death. In fact, subjects on chlorthalidone, who had lower levels of potassium, had the lowest incidence of cardiac deaths. In addition, there were fewer, not more, deaths among patients with abnormal exercise stress tests treated with high doses of diuretics. This debate can be clarified by reviewing the data in Table X.

It has been recognized for years that an abnormal ECG dramatically *increases* the risk of mortality from cardiovascular disease in hypertensive individuals. But, in the UC group in MRFIT (the group who received diuretics but in smaller dosages) patients who had *abnormal* ECGs experienced a *lower* mortality than those with normal ECGs, clearly an aberrant finding (17.7/1,000 compared to 20.7/1,000). The special intervention group, or those patients receiving higher doses of diuretics, showed a ratio of about 2:1 in CHD mortality between those with abnormal ECGs and those with normal ECGs (29.2/1,000 compared to 15.8/1,000). This is similar to findings in other studies. It was the *unusual* finding of a lower mortality in subjects from the UC cohort, with abnormal ECGs, that distorted the ratio and suggested an apparent diuretic-induced increase in mortality. Unfortunately, little effort was made to examine these data carefully or to popularize subsequent data from this study since at that time it was fashionable to consider newer drugs and to abandon the older ones.

Other Data on Hypokalemia and Arrhythmias

A small study of 21 subjects who had been carefully selected because of severe hypokalemia (K < 3.0 mEq/L) resulting from the

Table X. The Multiple Risk Factor Intervention Trial (MRFIT)[69,70]*

Statement From the Paper:
*A subgroup of patients with abnormal electrocardiograms (ECGs) at base-line in the special intervention group (SI) had a higher coronary heart disease (CHD) mortality than a comparable group in the usual care (UC) group. *Possibility that SI subjects responded adversely to MRFIT intervention* (i.e., higher dose of diuretics).

Evidence Against This Statement:

Hypertensives	CHD Deaths Mortality Rate/1,000	
	SI	UC
With abnormal resting ECGs	29.2	17.7*
With normal resting ECGs	15.8	20.7

Subjects with abnormal ECGs in the UC group had an unusually low CHD mortality. Had the ratio of about 2:1 found in other studies (mortality in subjects with abnormal compared to normal ECGs) held, this UC group would have noted an approximate 40/1,000 mortality. (see text)
In addition, SI subjects with abnormal exercise stress tests had a lower CHD mortality than UC subjects with abnormal stress tests. These were the patients who most probably had ischemic heart disease.

use of high-dose diuretics reported an increase in arrhythmias in 7 patients.[72] But many subsequent studies in subjects with and without LVH before and after exercise have failed to confirm these data—despite the use of dosages of HCTZ of 100 mg/gd.[73] In the SHEP[47,65] and Treatment of Mild Hypertension Study (TOMHS)[58] trials, no increase in ectopy was noted in diuretic treated subjects on continuous 24-hour Holter monitoring pre- and post-therapy.

One retrospective case control study did suggest an increase in sudden death with high-dose diuretics compared to lower dose diuretics given with potassium-sparing agents.[74] The case and control subjects differed considerably, and the study suffered from many of the flaws of any case control review. There has not been an increase in sudden death in any of the long-term diuretic-based clinical trials in both middle-aged and older individuals. Another retrospective nonrandomized study suggested an increase in CHD deaths with diuretics and ß-blockers.[75] This study suffers from the same methodological flaws as other case control studies and results are inconsistent with other carefully controlled trials. None of these latter trials had suggested an increase in CHD mortality with ß-blockers.

Many physicians are now ready to move on, to put in perspective the pronouncements about the alleged cardiotoxicity of diuretics and to look for the most acceptable way to use these agents. But for about the past 10 years, a great deal of effort, energy, and money was expended to wean physicians away from their use and in criticizing the JNC recommendations that diuretics continue to be used as initial therapy. *Myths about the dangers of diuretics have begun to disappear just as the terms "benign" and "mild" hypertension have become clarified. In years to come these speculations will be referred to as the errors of yesteryear, along with the "don't treat—it won't do any good" philosophy, etc.*

Renin Profiling—A Theory With Limited Clinical Usefulness

The advice that renin profiling was necessary for an accurate diagnosis, to predict outcome, or to determine specific therapy in the management of hypertension helped to confuse physicians for many years. This represents yet another example of attempting to apply a theory to the practice of medicine that, while appearing quite logical, has rarely helped the clinician in his or her approach to treatment.

It was repeatedly emphasized in the 1960's–1980's by a group of well known investigators that plasma renin levels should be an integral part of the diagnostic evaluation.[75a] While the importance of the renin-angiotensin-aldosterone system is well recognized as a contributory etiologic factor in hypertension, most treatment decisions can be made without evaluating components of this system.

JNC IV[54]—A Change in the Treatment Algorithm

In 1988 lifestyle changes or nonpharmacologic approaches to therapy were again recommended as initial approaches to treatment. However, the recommendations for therapy were changed; CCBs and ACE inhibitors were added to diuretics and ß-blockers as appropriate initial therapy (Table IX). The CCBs and ACE inhibitors had proven effective in reducing blood pressure and were reasonably well tolerated. There were some suggestions that these agents might have some specific beneficial properties over and above their blood pressure lowering effects, but there were still no long-term morbidity or mortality outcome data available (they had not been used in any of the long-term treatment trials).

JNC V[46]

Between 1988 and 1992 additional well controlled randomized 3–5 year studies that used diuretics with and without a potassium-sparing component as initial therapy or compared diuretics to ß-blockers, confirmed that both cerebrovascular and cardiovascular morbidity and mortality were reduced by treatment in middle-aged and elderly subjects[51] (Fig. 5). Not only were benefits noted in subjects with systolic and diastolic hypertension but also in those with isolated systolic hypertension.[47] Therapy with these agents, alone, or in combination, not only reduced strokes and CHD events but also the occurrence of LVH and CHF as well as progression from less severe to more severe disease.[31] Data were still not available with other medications. One might question the reasons for this lack of data since in 1992 CCBs and ACE

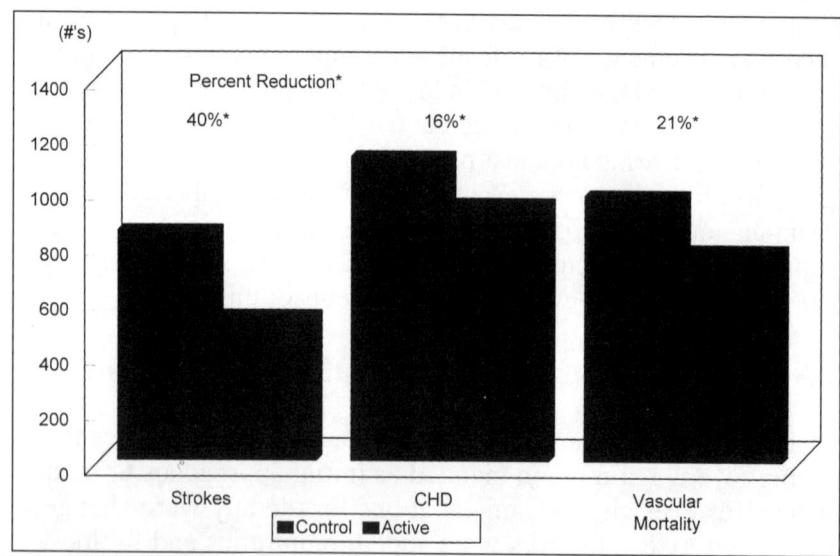

Figure 5. Effect of antihypertensive drug treatment on coronary heart disease, strokes and vascular mortality in seventeen 3- to 5-year clinical trials.[51]
*Highly statistically significant. CHD = coronary heart disease

inhibitors had been available for more than 10–15 years. There may have been the perception that it wasn't necessary to do any long-term studies since physicians were prescribing them anyway in more than 50% of hypertensive patients without long-term outcome data.

Based on new outcome data with diuretics and ß-blockers, the JNC in 1993 recommended them as preferred initial therapy. Calcium channel blockers, ACE inhibitors, α-blockers, and α-ß-blockers were suggested as possible alternative therapy (Table IX). This was a reasonable recommendation based on the available evidence. There were, however, many physicians who disagreed with these recommendations—the report was widely criticized. JNC V was characterized as a document that took a step forward (defining stages of hypertension and the importance of systolic blood pressure) and a step backward (classifying the *most frequently* prescribed antihypertensive drugs, the ACE inhibitors and CCBs as *alternative* initial therapy). Subsequent information, since 1993, however, appears to have vindicated the JNC recommendations.

Numerous clinical trials are now in progress with the newer antihypertensive agents; but we will have to await the results of these ongoing studies before a definate decision can be made that medications other than diuretics and ß-blockers have equal or more favorable effects on cardiovascular morbidity and mortality. While awaiting these data, the ACE inhibitors, angiotensin II receptor antagonists and CCBs, as well as the other agents, should be used in special situations or where diuretics or ß-blockers are contraindicated. These indications are reviewed in detail elsewhere and listed in Table XI.[76,77]

Based on studies over the past 5 years, it would appear that the ACE inhibitors and probably the angiotensin II receptor antagonists have a special role in the treatment of patients with diabetic nephropathy and CHF. It should be emphasized, however, that the benefits of ACE inhibitors in both CHF and nephropathy patients have usually been achieved when these medications are used along with a diuretic. Results have been reported and discussed as ACE inhibitor trials; in fact, these have been trials of multidrug therapy. It is highly possible that the use of agents that block the renin-angiotensin-aldosterone system at various sites will result in a reduction of morbidity and mortality in long-term trials with hypertensive subjects. Better results will probably be obtained, however, when these medications are used with a diuretic.

Table XI. Some Special Indications for Specific Classes of Antihypertensive Medications[75,76]

1. CHF	a) ACE inhibitor or A_{11} receptor antagonist (usually with a directic) b) α_1-ß-Blocker (Carvedilol) plus diuretics and digitalis
2. Diabetes mellitus–type I with nephropathy probably also in type II	ACE inhibitor (with small doses diuretic) Probably A_{II}
3. Angina	a) ß-Blockers (non-ISA) b) Selected CCBs
4. Postmyocardial infarction	a) ß-Blockers (non-ISA) b) ACE inhibitor c) α_1-ß-Blocker (Carvedilol)
5. Migraine headaches	a) ß-Blockers b) Verapamil c) Diltiazem
6. Atrial fibrillation	ß-Blockers (non-ISA)
7. Prostatic hypertrophy	α-Blockers

AII = angiotensin II receptor antagonist
ACE = angiotensin-converting enzyme
CHF = congestive heart failure
ISA = intrinsic sympathomimetic activity

Data thus far do not appear to justify advocating CCB therapy (especially the shorter-acting agents) as initial treatment except perhaps in the elderly patient with isolated systolic hypertension. The question must be asked in 1997, Why are these still the most popular antihypertensive medications—promotional activities or scientific data?

The Calcium Channel Blocker Debate

The issue of the safety of CCBs in hypertensive subjects provides another example of possible misinterpretation or over-interpretation of suggestive but not definitive data. Following the reports of Psaty,[78] and Pahor,[79] and the review article by Furberg,[80] the news media proclaimed that the use of these agents may not only increase heart attack risk and heart failure but may also increase the incidence of cancer.[81] There are strong suggestions that the use of the shorter acting CCBs may increase CHD risk and do not have the expected effect of slowing down progression of the atherogenic process. Several of the studies reporting this were, however, retrospective case control studies and suffered from the same design problems as the "diuretics increase the risk of sudden death" reviews. One prospective controlled study comparing a dihydropyridine CCB to a diuretic did demonstrate an increase in new onset angina in the CCB subjects compared to those treated with HCTZ.[82] As noted, a recent nonrandomized trial using a longer acting CCB reported a reduction in strokes and severe arrhythmias but, the design of this trial is flawed in many areas.[83] We should await more definitive data regarding the benefits and risks of the longer acting CCBs before reaching conclusions regarding their safety in hypertensive subjects—the longer acting agents should continue to be used in special situations and physicians should be careful not to react to headlines or emotional presentations.

It may very well be that there are problems with the use of some CCBs and they will not live up to their "promotional" promises, but a wait and see attitude is probably justified in 1997. Based on available data, however, the use of the shorter acting agents in this class of drugs should be avoided.

The CCB debate is another example of an over reaction to preliminary, hypothesis-generating data. Industry and "physician advocate" reactions to these initial papers was dramatic in strong contrast to the muted or nonexistent response to the same kind of case control retrospective analyses that proclaimed the dangers of diuretics. There was no large constituency for these latter agents. In contrast to the CCBs however, there were data on long-term benefits when diuretics were used.

Combination Therapy

The Chinese had an early answer to therapy which circumvented SC. A capsule, which included small amounts of reserpine, potassium, chlorothiazide, thiamine, calcium, magnesium, and B6, was reported to clear up the blood pressure in 100% of patients whom we now classify as stage I or II, and more than 85% of those with more severe hypertension (Table XII). If the patients failed to respond to this initial therapy, a more potent combination of these ingredients was given, and hydralazine and some guanethidine were added.

   Combination therapy with small doses of 2 different drugs is being accepted once again as a reasonable treatment approach to achieve blood pressure lowering with fewer side effects. Combinations were widely used in the 1960s and 1970s—reserpine/thiazide, reserpine/hydralazine/thiazide, etc. At present effective combinations of thiazide-ß-blockers, thiazide-ACE inhibitors, thiazides and angiotensin II receptor blockers, and CCBs and ACE inhibitors are available. Two of these combinations, bisoprolol (a ß-blocker)/HCTZ (Ziac) and captopril (an ACE inhibitor)/HCTZ (Capozide) have been approved as initial therapy and are available for use. Recent studies have demonstrated that the ß-blocker/thiazide combination produces fewer side effects and has an equal or higher response rate than monotherapy with a CCB or ACE inhibitor. Betaxolol/HCTZ has also been approved but is not being marketed at present. An ACE inhibitor or angiotensin II receptor antagonist/diuretic combination or an

---

Table XII. Example of Chinese Approach to Multidrug Therapy for Hypertension

This capsule is a complex preparation consisting of rauwolfia alkaloid and other agents such as sedative, diuretic, and blood-potassium equilibrium salt. Each capsule contains:

Reserpine	0.03 mg	Promethiazine	2.1 mg
Potassium chloride	30 mg	Calcium lactate	1 mg
Hydrochlorothiazide	3.1 mg	Magnesium trisilicate	30 mg
Vitamin B1	1 mg	Vitamin B6	1mg
Chloriazepoxide	1 mg	Dibazolum	10 mg

Based on the reports of 8 major hospitals, this capsule can be extensively used in the treatment of hypertension at various stages. When given orally, it will relieve the subjective symptoms of the patient. Clinical experiments on 300 cases have proved that this medicine has a conspicuous therapeutic effect on primary hypertension at various stages, with the effective rate being 100% for the first stage, 95.6% for the second, and 89.7% for the third.

Minchin Pharmaceutical Factor, China National Medicines & Health Products Import & Export Corporation, Fujian Branch

ACE/CCB combination also lower blood pressure to a greater extent than monotherapy, with fewer adverse reactions—none of these, however, have as yet been approved as initial therapy.

One may look back 10 years from now and wonder why so many physicians had taken the strong position that combination therapy represented "shot gun" medicine and that this approach did not "individualize" therapy and should not be used as initial treatment (see below).

Public Health Aspects of Hypertension Control

What has happened to hypertension control through the years? We have made progress in disseminating the message that hypertension is not a benign disease—it took quite a long time. As late as the 1970s fewer than 50% of people with hypertension knew they had it, and a large number of those who knew about it were not being treated or controlled. Fewer than 15% of all hypertensives were being controlled at levels below 160/90 mm Hg, a goal of therapy that has since been adjusted to 140/90 mm Hg.

It was estimated that almost 20% of all people in the U. S. had diastolic blood pressures of 95 mm Hg or higher. In the 1970s and 1980s an elevated systolic blood pressure was not often considered when defining risk or in evaluating results of treatment programs, despite data that it probably represents a more important risk factor than the diastolic pressure. This misconception has finally been clarified by excellent follow-up data. From 1972 to 1981 the number of people who were unaware that they had

Table XIII. Hypertension Awareness, Treatment, and Control Rates[77]*			
	1976–1980[II]	1988-91	1988–1991[III]
Aware (%)	51%	73%	68.4%
Treated (%)	31%	55%	53.6%
Controlled (%)	10%	29%	27.4%
*Defined as 140/90 mm Hg or more on 1 occasion or reported to be currently taking antihypertensive medication.			
National Health and Nutrition Examination Surveys I, II, and III (phase I and II).			

hypertension decreased dramatically. National statistics from the National Hygiene and Nutritional Survey (NHANES) III in 1991 show that 73% of all people with elevated blood pressure in the U.S. are aware that they have it if 140 / 90 mm Hg or higher is considered as the definition of hypertension (Table XIII).

The pattern of patients under therapy and control in the 1970s and 1980s is also of interest (Table XIVa and XIVb). The percentage of people being treated and under control was considerably higher in the late 1970s and 1980s in some areas reported in this summary because of large-scale screening and treatment programs. For example, the number of patients under control increased dramatically from 11% to 61%, and from 43% to 72% in the 10-year period between surveys in Chicago and Westchester County respectively.[85]

In the most recent NHANES study only 53.6% of people with blood pressures > 140/90 mm Hg are being treated and, if 140/90 mm Hg is used as a criterion of control, only 27.4% of the total hypertensives or only about 50% of those on therapy are actually being treated to goal levels (Table XIV). We have a long way to go to improve these results.

Why are so many people not being treated effectively despite abundant data 1) defining hypertension as a cardiovascular risk factor, 2) the very clear evidence of benefit from blood pressure lowering and, 3) the availability of effective and well tolerated therapy?

The myth that hypertension was not significant or important has been refuted. The number of visits to doctors for hypertension has increased dramatically, and in recent years hypertension has become the most common reason that adults see physicians in the U.S. There are still many physicians, however, who are not treating patients with less severe hypertension or to goal pressures of below 140/90 mm Hg. An editorial/comment in *American Family Physician* in 1996, highlights one of the problems:

> "Simply stated"
>
> The strategic targets for our attention
> in primary care are patients with severe
> hypertension (diastolic pressures over
> 110 mm Hg), elderly patients, those with
> diabetes, patients who are at high risk for
> stroke, and those with known heart disease.[86]

Table XIVa. Status of Hypertension Control

	National Heart Survey (1960–1962)	Chicago (1967–1971)	Atlanta (1970)	HDFP Study (1973–1974)	Westchester County, NY (1975)
# Examined	6,672	22,929	6,012	158,906	11,534
% With DBP > 95 mm Hg	15.0	20.0	23.0	13.2	23.0
% Unaware of high BP	43.0	59.0	19.0	25.0	21.0
% With high BP being treated	36.0	25.0	57.0	54.0	60.0
% With high BP under control	16.0	11.0	36.0	38.0	43.0

Table XIVb. Status of Hypertension Control

	Chicago (1977)	Minneapolis (1980–1981)	Chicago (1982)	Westchester County, NY (1981–1982)	Ontario Canada (1981–1982)
# Examined	117,954	1,656	56,078*	35,580*	2,735
% With DBP > 95 mm Hg	13.2	14.0	?*	?*	?
% Unaware of high BP	11.9	13.0	6.0	4.0	7.0
% With high BP being treated	76.1	76.1	69.0	87.0	92.0
% With high BP under control	59.3	59.3	61.0	72.0	70.0

*Includes unknown number of repeat examinations of different criteria for elevated diastolic blood pressure

BP = blood pressure

DBP = diastolic blood pressure

These comments, reminiscent of statements 30–40 years ago, were addressed to family practitioners and completely ignore data from numerous studies that report benefits of therapy in middle-age subjects as well as the elderly, and in patients with diastolic blood pressures well below 110 mm Hg and without heart disease. Physicians are still being confused by beliefs that should have been dispelled years ago. This confusion is just one reason why some practitioners are still reluctant to treat many patients who should be treated.

In addition to the fact that some physicians are still reluctant to lower pressures to a reasonable goal of below 140/90 mm Hg, there are many patients who are not convinced that therapy is necessary or important enough to warrant continuing medication over their lifetime. Titration of dosages of medication or the adding or subtracting of different medications is often troublesome to a busy practitioner and to patients who are unable to see immediate benefit from these actions. The message of prevention of complications of hypertension must be reemphasized. The promotional negativism that "we haven't achieved a reduction in CHD events" with those "older" drugs and that "only this new and usually more expensive drug will do the job" must somehow be tempered. Newer agents may have advantages and be well worth the increased cost; they should be used in appropriate situations. Studies may prove them to be superior to present therapy. It is also possible that changing other risk factors will result in better outcome, but we need not wait 4–7 years to find out. We must reinforce the strong and correct message now—*blood pressure lowering by itself has been highly effective in reducing morbidity and mortality*. We can proceed from this fact and hope that we can do even better, but we should not confuse the practitioner or patients—we should concentrate on a scientifically valid message—and the relative simplicity in managing a majority of patients with hypertension.

Patient Education

Lip service is often given to patient education, but how many physician's offices have more than the sketchiest of educational material on hypertension in their treatment or consultation rooms—-despite the availability of numerous booklets, available free-of-charge from the National High Blood Pressure Information Center, 120/80 National Institutes of Health,

Bethesda, MD 20892, and the American Heart Association.

Reading material in itself is not the answer to improving the percentage of hypertensive patients under control, but it is one approach that helps.

Where Do We Go From Here?

There are several newer antihypertensive agents available, but at present, we have no data that their use will decrease morbidity and mortality to as great or greater degree than older medications. One of the newer classes of drugs is the angiotensin II receptor antagonists. At least 3 or 4 more medications in this class will be available within the next year or two. Do these agents represent a major advance in treatment? As monotherapy, the angiotensin II receptor antagonists are probably as efffective as the ACE inhibitors. In many cases, a diuretic must be added to achieve goal pressures. The combination is highly effective and makes good physiologic sense. These newer drugs do not cause a cough, which may be noted in as many as 20% of patients on an ACE inhibitor.[87]

The promotional messages with these newer agents represent another interesting "flip flop" of confusing information in the ongoing story of hypertension treatment. When the ACE inhibitors were marketed, we were told that, as a result of the action of the ACE inhibitor, not only was the generation of angiotensin II interfered with, but the degradation or breakdown of bradykinin was prevented. Angiotensin-converting enzyme inhibitors, therefore, lowered blood pressure by 2 mechanisms—increased bradykinin (and prostaglandins) and a decrease in the generation of angiotensin II and aldosterone. The double action was reported with enthusiasm. With the introduction of angiotensin II receptor antagonists, which do not have an effect on the bradykinin cascade, we are now told that excess bradykinin may not have been a good thing after all—that's why patients had a cough or developed angioedema. It may be that these newer agents will be more useful than the ACE inhibitors, but messages appear to change to fit the treatment of the moment.

A new α-ß-blocker, carvedilol, has also been approved for therapy in hypertension. This agent has potent antioxidant properties and has also been shown to reduce morbidity and mortality in patients with heart failure who had not satisfactorily responded to ACE inhibitor, diuretic, and digitalis therapy.

Renin inhibitors are also being studied, as are medications that either augment the effects or prevent the degradation of endothelium relaxing factor nitric oxide (NO). If an orally effective stimulator of NO production could be developed, this could represent an advance in treatment.

Vasopressor antagonists are being studied again after having been ignored for about 20 years. Endopeptidase inhibitors that prevent the breakdown of atrial natriuretic factor, a factor which increases sodium excretion and lowers blood pressure, might also prove useful. Some investigators also believe that if insulin sensitivity can be increased, blood pressure might be better controlled.

Finally, several genes have been identified that may play a causative role in hypertension. Mutations of these genes have been identified in certain susceptible populations. The potential for gene therapy in hypertension is one that will be watched with interest but is probably a long way from clinical use.

The Challenge

The challenge now is to convince more physicians that treatment is worthwhile and that it is not enough to say "Yes, I treat all of my patients with hypertension." Treatment must be pursued to a goal of 140/90 mm Hg or below. This may require a renewed and perhaps slightly different approach than has been used in the past, especially in certain populations groups. Recent studies have again suggested that even subjects with stage I hypertension will benefit from treatment.[58] Patient compliance or adherence to a treatment program is important, but the role of physicians remains paramount. *We will not see further improvement in outcome until more physicians become convinced that treatment does not just mean giving out medication.* Data indicate that about 80%–85% of all hypertensive patients can be treated to normotensive levels with available therapy.[88]

SUMMARY

We have come a long way since the era of rigid low-salt diets and mutilative surgery, and from the time when many physicians believed that hypertension was a natural feature of aging and that there was little we could do about it. Many of the misconceptions and myths have been clarified and the heroics of the pioneers in hypertension treatment and their patients have resulted in significant advancements in our concept and implementation of therapy. The era of modern-day therapy has brought with it some major treatment successes. Stroke mortality has decreased by about 58% since the start of the NHBPEP in 1972 and the demonstration that lowering of blood pressure would reduce morbidity and mortality. All of this benefit is not, however, just the result of better management of hypertension. We smoke less, we exercise more, we eat less fatty foods, and we are more aware of health in general, but management of hypertension has a lot to do with it, since about 75%–80% of all strokes occur in hypertensive individuals.

There has also been a 50% decrease in CHD. Of course, this improvement is also not just the result of better management of hypertension. As noted, people smoke less and exercise more, and the existence of coronary care units, thrombolytic therapy, and surgical procedures have helped to reduce CHD death rates. Better control of hypertension, however, has had to have an impact on this disease.

We have learned since the 1920s that the kidney is not the cause of all hypertension. We now know that death is not an inevitable outcome of hypertension. We no longer have to deprive people of the enjoyment of life when we treat their high blood pressure. We should no longer ignore even slight elevations of blood pressure. And we should remember the story of Franklin D. Roosevelt and the poor results of treatment in the 1930s and 1940s before effective antihypertensive medications were available. Above all, we should look carefully at new pronouncements and recommendations for treatment and be guided by data and science, not speculations and theories. These may generate useful hypotheses but should not be used as indications for treatment changes.

REFERENCES

1. Scott RW. Clinical Blood Pressure. In: Tice F. *Practice of Medicine.* 1946;6:93–114.
2. Weiss E. *Psychosomatic Medicine.* 1939;1:180.
3. Bruenn HG. Clinical notes on the illness and death of President Franklin D. Roosevelt. *Ann Int Med.* 1970;72:579–591.
4. Kempner W. Treatment of hypertensive vascular disease with rice diet. *Am J Med.* 1948;4:545–577.
5. Keith NM, Wagener HP, Barker NW. Some different types of essential hypertension: Their cause and prognosis. *Am J Med Sci.* 1939;197:332–343.
6. Bechgaard P. Arterial hypertension, follow-up study of 1,000 hypertensives. *Acta Scandinavia.* 1946 (suppl 172).
7. Smithwick R. The effects of sympathectomy upon the mortality and survival rates of patients with hypertensive cardiovascular disease. In: Bell ET (ed). *Hypertension*, Minnesota Press. 1951:429–457.
8. Peet MM. Results of subdiaphragmatic splanchnicectomy for arterial hypertension. *N Engl J Med.* 1947;236:270–276.
9. Freis ED, Wilkins RW. Effect of pentaquine in patients with hypertension. *Proc Soc Exp Biol & Med.* 1947;64:731–736.
10. Page IH, Taylor RD. Pyrogens in the treatment of malignant hypertension. *Mod Concepts Cardiovasc Dis.* 1949;18:51–52.
11. Moyer JH. Cardiovascular and renal hemodynamic response to reserpine (Serpasil) and clinical results using this agent for treatment of hypertension. *Ann NY Acad Sci.* 1954;59:82–94.
12. Moser M. Evaluation of drug therapy of hypertension. *NY State J Med.* 1955;55:1999.
13. Hines EA. The thiocyanates in the treatment of hypertensive disease. *Med Clin N Am.* 1946;30:869–877.
14. Freis ED, Stanton JR. Clinical evaluation of veratrum viride in treatment of essential hypertension. *Am Heart J.* 1948;36:723–738.
15. Schroeder HM, Perry H, Mitchell JR, et al. Chemical con-

trol of hypertension. *Science.* 1952;116:528.

16. Perry HM, Schroeder HA. Syndrome simulating collagen disease caused by hydralazine (Apresoline). *JAMA.* 1954;154:670–673.

17. Moser M. Walters M, Master AM, et al. Chemical blockade of the sympathetic nervous system in essential hypertension (experience with 688A). *Arch Int Med.* 1952;89:708.

18. Moser M, Macauley AK, Granzen R, et al. Drug therapy of hypertension II. Experience with reserpine, apresoline, ansolysen, ecolid and mecamylamine. *NY State J Med.* 1956;56: 2487–2497.

19. Moser M, Mattingly TW. Critical evaluation of drug therapy of hypertension. *Postgrad Med.* 1955;17:351.

20. Restall PA, Smirk FH. The treatment of high blood pressure with hexamethonium iodide. *New Zealand Med J.* 1950;49:206–209.

21. Freis ED, Rose JC, Partenope A, et al. The hemodynamic effect of hypotensive drugs in man. III. Hexamethonium. *J Clin Invest.* 1953; 32:1285–1298.

22. Freis ED. Hydralazine in pharmacology and clinical application. In: Moyer J and Brest AN (eds). *Hypertension—Recent Advances*, Lea & Febiger, Philadelphia, PA. 1961:291–295.

23. Schroeder HA. Treatment of Hypertension by Hyphex. In: Schroeder HA (ed). *Hypertensive Diseases*, Lea & Febiger, Philadelphia, PA. 1953:474–540.

24. Perrera GA. Hypertensive Vascular Disease: Description and Natural History. *J Chron Dis.* 1955;1:33.

25. Freis ED, Wanko A, Wilson IM, et al. Treatment of hypertension with chlorothiazide (Diuril). *JAMA.* 1958;166:137.

26. Moser M, Macaulay AC. Chlorothiazide as an adjunct in the treatment of hypertension. *Am J Cardiol.* 1959;3:214.

27. Page IH. The renin angiotensin pressor system. In: Bell ET (ed). *Hypertension*, Minnesota Press. 1957:66.

28. Moser M. A decade of progress in the management of hypertension. *Hypertens.* 1983;5:808–813.

29. Moyer JH, Heider C, Pevey K, et al. The effect of treatment on the vascular deterioration associated with hypertension, with particular emphasis on renal function. *Am J Med.* 1958;24:177.

30. Goldring W, Chasis H. Antihypertensive Drug Therapy. In: Ingelfinger FG (ed). *Controversies in Internal Medicine*, W.B.

Saunders & Co., Philadelphia, PA. 1966:83–91.

31. Moser M, Hebert P. Prevention of disease progression, left ventricular hypertrophy and congestive heart failure in the hypertension treatment trials. *J Am Coll Cardiol.* 1996;27(5):1214–1218.

32. Pickering G. On the management of patients with hypertension. In: Moser M and Goldman AG. *Hypertensive Vascular Disease*, J.B. Lippincott Co., Philadelphia, PA. 1967.

33. Friedberg CK. *Diseases of the Heart*, W.B. Saunders & Co., Philadelphia, PA. 1966.

34. Tibbets. *Br Med J.* 1950;2:1452.

35. Veterans Administration Cooperative Study Group on Antihypertensive Agents. Effects of treatment on morbidity in hypertension. Results in patients with diastolic blood pressures averaging 115 through 129 mm Hg. *JAMA.* 1967;202:1028–1034.

36. U.S. Public Health Service Hospitals Cooperative Study Group. Treatment of mild hypertension. Results of a ten-year intervention trial. *Circ Res.* 1977;40(suppl 1):98–105.

37. Hypertension Detection and Follow-up Program Cooperative Group. Five-year findings of the Hypertension Detection and Follow-up Program. I. Reduction in mortality of persons with high blood pressure, including mild hypertension. *JAMA.* 1979;242:2562–2571.

38. Report of the Joint National Committee on Detection, Evaluation and Treatment of High Blood Pressure. *JAMA.* 1977; 237:255–261.

39. Australian National Blood Pressure Management Committee. The Australian therapeutic trial in mild hypertension. *Lancet.* 1980;1:1261–1267.

40. MRC Working Party. Medical Research Council trial of treatment of mild hypertension: Principal results. *Br Med J.* 1985;291:97–104.

41. Moser M. Low-dose diuretic therapy for hypertension. *Clin Ther.* 1986;8(5);554–562.

42. Veterans Administration Cooperative Study Group on Antihypertensive Agents. Low doses vs. standard dose of reserpine, a randomized double-blind multiclinic trial in patients taking chlorthalidone. *JAMA.* 1982;248:2471–2477.

43. Veterans Administration Cooperative Study Group on Antihypertensive Agents. Captopril: Evaluation of low doses,

twice daily doses and the addition of diuretic for the treatment of mild to moderate hypertension. *Clin Sci.* 1982;63(suppl 8):4435– 4455.

44. McFate Smith W. Mild Hypertension: To Treat or Not To Treat. *Ann NY Acad Sci.* 1978;304:466.

45. Krishan I, Moser M. Treatment of Hypertension 1981. In: Conn HF (ed). *Current Therapy*, W.B. Saunders & Co., Philadelphia, PA. 1982:200–206.

46. Report of the Joint National Committee on Detection, Evaluation and Treatment of High Blood Pressure (JNC V). *Arch Int Med.* 1993;153:154–183.

47. SHEP Cooperative Research Group. Prevention of stroke by antihypertensive drug treatment in older persons with isolated systolic hypertension. *JAMA.* 1991;265:3255–3264.

48. Dahlof B, Lindholm LH, Hansson L, et al. Morbidity and mortality in the Swedish trial in old patients with hypertension (STOP-Hypertension). *Lancet.* 1991;338:1281–1285.

49. MRC Working Party. Medical Research Council trial of treatment of hypertension in older adults: Principal results. *Br Med J.* 1992;304:405–412.

50. Amery A, Birkenhager W, Brixko P, et al. Mortality and morbidity results from the European Working Party on High Blood Pressure in the Elderly Trial. *Lancet.* 1985;1:1349–1354.

51. Hebert P, Moser M, Mayer J, et al. Recent evidence on drug therapy of mild to moderate hypertension and decreased risk of coronary heart disease. *Arch Intern Med.* 1993;153:578–581.

52. Report of the Joint National Committee on Detection, Evaluation and Treatment of High Blood Pressure. *Arch Intern Med.* 1980;140:1280.

53. Report of the Joint National Committee on Detection, Evaluation and Treatment of High Blood Pressure. *Arch Intern Med.* 1984;144:1045–1057.

54. Report of the Joint National Committee on Detection, Evaluation and Treatment of High Blood Pressure. *Arch Intern Med.* 1988;148:1023–1038.

55. Moser M. Suppositions and speculations—their possible effects on treatment decisions in the management of hypertension. *Am Heart J.* 1989;118:1362–1369.

56. Lind L, Pollare T, Berne C. Long-term metabolic effects of antihypertensive drugs. *Am Heart J.* 1994;128:1177–1183.

57. Middeke M, Weisweiler P, Schwandt P, et al. Serum lipoprotein during antihypertensive therapy with beta blockers and diuretics: A controlled long-term comparative trial. *Clin Cardiol.* 1987;10:94–98.

58. Neaton JD, Grimm RH, Prineas RJ, et al for the Treatment of Mild Hypertension Study Research Group. Treatment of mild hypoertension study: Final results. *JAMA.* 1993;270:713–724.

59. Materson BJ, Reda DJ, Cushman WC, et al. Single-drug therapy for hypertension in men: A comparison of six antihypertensive agents with placebo. The Department of Veterans Affairs Cooperative Study Group on Antihypertensive Agents. *N Engl J Med.* 1993;328:914–921.

60. Zusman RM. Alternatives to traditional antihypertensive therapy (Editorial). *Hyperten*s. 1986;8:837–842.

61. McInnes GT, Yeo WW, Ramsey LE, et al. Cardiotoxicity and diuretics: Much speculation, little substance. *J Hyperten*s. 1992;10:317–335.

62. Houston MC. New insights and new approaches for the treatment of essential hypertension: Selection of therapy based on coronary heart disease risk factor analysis, hemodynamic profiles, quality of life, and subsets of hypertension. *Am Heart J.* 1989;117:911–949.

63. Freis ED. Critique of the clinical importance of diuretic-induced hypokalemia and elevated cholesterol levels. *Arch Intern Med.* 1989;149:2649–2658.

64. Moser M. Current hypertension management: Separating fact from fiction. *Cleveland Clin J Med.* 1993;60:27–37.

65. Curb JD, Pressel SL, Cutler JA, et al. Effect of diuretic-based antihypertensive treatment on cardiovascular disease risk in older diabetic patients with isolated systolic hypertension. *JAMA.* 1996;276:1886–1892.

66. Gurwitz GH, Bohn RL, Glynn RJ, et al. Antihypertensive drug therapy and the initiation of treatment for diabetes mellitus. *Ann Intern Med.* 1993;118:273–278.

67. Warram JH, Laffel LMB, Vasania P, et al. Excess mortality associated with diuretic therapy in diabetes mellitus. *Arch Intern Med.* 1991;151:1350–1356.

68. Pollare T, Lithell H, Berne C. A comparison of the effects of hydrochlorothiazide and captopril on glucose and lipid metabolism in patients with hypertension. *N Engl J Med.*

1989;321:868–873.

69. Multiple Risk Factor Intervention Trial Research Group. Risk factor changes and mortality results. *JAMA.* 1982;248:1465–1477.

70. Multiple Risk Factor Intervention Trial Research Group. Exercise electrocardiogram and coronary heart disease mortality in the Multiple Risk Factor Intervention Trial. *Am J Cardiol.* 1985;55:16–24.

71. Moser M. Clinical trials and their effect on medical therapy. The Multiple Risk Factor Intervention Trial. *Am Heart J.* 1984; 107:616–618.

72. Holland OB, Nixon JV, Kuhnert I. Diuretic-induced ventricular ectopic activity. *Am J Med.* 1981;770:762–768.

73. Papademetriou V, et al. Thiazide therapy is not a cause of arrhythmia in patients with systemic hypertension. *Arch Intern Med.* 1988;148:1272–1276.

74. Siscovick DS, Raghunathan TE, Psaty BM, et al. Diuretic therapy for hypertension and the risk of primary cardiac arrest. *N Engl J Med.* 1994;330:1852–1857.

75. Hoes AW, Grobbee DE, Hubsen J, et al. Diuretics, ß-blockers and the risk of sudden cardiac death in hypertension patients. *Ann Intern Med.* 1995;123:481–487.

75a. Brunner HR, Sealey JE, Laragh JH. Renin as a risk factor in essential hypertension. *Am J Med.* 1973;55:295.

76. Moser M. *Hyperten*sion. In: Rakel R (ed). *Conn's Current Therapy*, W.B. Saunders & Co., Philadelphia, PA. 1995:263–280.

77. Moser M. Management of hypertension, Part II. *Am Fam Phys.* 1966;53(8):2553–2560.

78. Psaty BM, Heckbert SR, Koepsell TD, et al. The risk of myocardial infarction associated with antihypertensive drug therapies. *JAMA.* 1995;274:620–625.

79. Pahor M, Guralnik JM, Corti MC, et al. Long-term survival and use of antihypertensive medications in older persons. *J Am Geriatrics Soc.* 1995;43:1191–1197.

80. Furberg CD, Psaty BM, Myers SV. Nifedipine dose related increase in mortality in patients with coronary heart disease. *Circulation.* 1995;92:1326–1331.

81. Pahor M, Guralnik JM, Salive ME, et al. Do calcium channel blockers increase the risk of cancer? *Am J Hyperten.* 1996;9:695–699.

82. Borhani NO, Mancini M, Borhani PA, et al. Final outcome results of the Multicenter Isradipine Diuretic Atherosclerosis Study (MIDAS). *JAMA*. 1996;276:785–791.

83. Gorg L, Zhang W, Zhu Y, et al. Shanghai Trial of Nifedipine in the Elderly (STONE). *J Hyperten*. 1996;14(10):1237–1245.

84. Burt V, Cutler J, Higgins M. Trends in the prevalence, awareness, treatment and control of hypertension in the adult U.S. population: Data from the Health Examination Surveys, 1960–1991. *Hypertens*. 1995;26:60–69.

85. Moser M. The National High Blood Pressure Education Program and Clinical Trials: Two decades of progress in the management of hypertension—*Hypertension Update II, IV*. 1985:46.

86. Kopes-Kerr CP. Hypertension and heart disease; How much is enough? *Am Fam Phys*. 1996;53(7):2274–2275.

87. Simon SR, Black HR, Moser M, et al. Cough and ACE inhibitors. *Arch Intern Med*. 1992;152:1698–1700.

88. Moser M, Okin P, Grollett K. Long term management of hypertension. private practice experience. *NY State J Med*. 1980;80:1102.